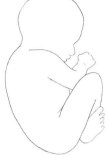

"An inspired and essential guide to creating the birth you desire! *The Doula's Guide to Empowering Your Birth* offers a golden opportunity to have your own personal, experienced doula guide you to an understanding of the many choices you have for you and your baby in birth and beyond. Lindsey Bliss, an experienced and wise doula, has witnessed birth in many ways and in these pages she provides the tips and wisdom you need to prepare for a safe, empowered, powerful, and truly memorable birth."

> —Debra Pascali-Bonaro, doula, doula trainer, creator of the Pain to Power childbirth program, and co-author of *Orgasmic Birth*

"Lindsey Bliss is an exceptional woman with years of life experience as the mother of seven children and hands-on experience as a doula who has dedicated her life to serving new mothers in both prosperous and underserved communities. *The Doula's Guide to Empowering Your Birth* translates medical language into plain English and explains the many choices available to you, so that you can be empowered in your birth."

> —Elizabeth Bachner, owner, midwife, and clinic director, GraceFull birthing center, Los Angeles

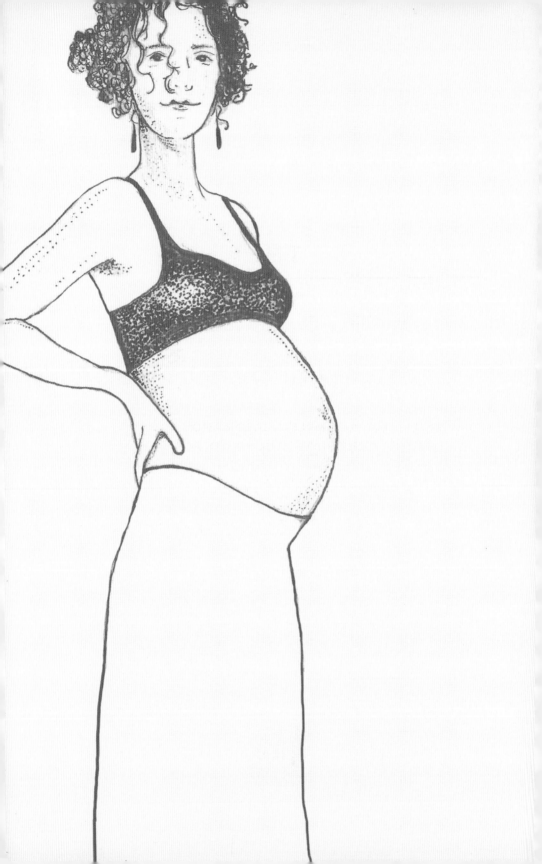

THE
DOULA'S GUIDE
TO EMPOWERING
YOUR BIRTH

A COMPLETE LABOR AND CHILDBIRTH COMPANION FOR PARENTS-TO-BE

LINDSEY BLISS

HARVARD
COMMON
PRESS

© 2018 Quarto Publishing Group USA Inc.
Text © Lindsey Bliss
Illustrations © Stephanie Lawson

First Published in 2018 by The Harvard Common Press, an imprint of The Quarto Group, 100 Cummings Center, Suite 265-D, Beverly, MA 01915, USA.
T (978) 282-9590 F (978) 283-2742
QuartoKnows.com

The Harvard Common Press titles are also available at discount for retail, wholesale, promotional, and bulk purchase. For details, contact the Special Sales Manager by email at specialsales@quarto.com or by mail at The Quarto Group, Attn: Special Sales Manager, 401 Second Avenue North, Suite 310, Minneapolis, MN 55401, USA.

22 21 20 19 18   2 3 4 5

ISBN: 978-1-55832-895-2

Library of Congress Cataloging-in-Publication Data is available

Design: Debbie Berne
Illustration: Stepha Lawson @thelanguageofbirth
www.languageofbirth.com

Printed in China

The information in this book is for educational purposes only. It is not intended to replace the advice of a physician or medical practitioner. Please see your health-care provider before beginning any new health program.

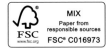

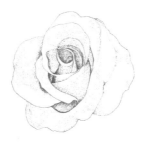

For my family and all of the families who have allowed
me to be a part of their childbearing journeys.

CONTENTS

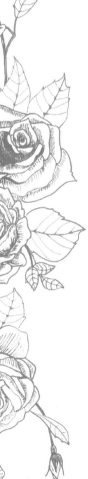

PART ONE

Your Pregnancy

INTRODUCTION

"You cannot use someone else's fire. You can only use your own. And
in order to do that, you must first be willing to believe that you have it."
—Audre Lorde

Are you pregnant and left with a bunch of burning questions? Do you
lack nonjudgmental support from your friends, family, and/or partner?
Are you afraid to give birth? We are inundated with media depictions of
childbirth as a fear-filled emergency event with an epic water breaking
scene and an explosive delivery with lots of screaming. In this book, I am
going to challenge this cultural conditioning and show you that childbirth can be a beautiful and transformative journey.

Countless friends have said to me, "After the birth of my first child,
I kept thinking, I wish someone had told me about this possibility," or
"I wish I had known about that fact." This book is based on my passionate
belief that it is time to restore the power of giving birth to its rightful
owner: *you*, the birthing person. As an experienced birth doula who
has seen more than 250 births over my eight-year career, and as the
mother of seven kids (including two sets of twins), I want to share with
parents-to-be all the possibilities out there for making their birthing
experiences their own. It is your body, your birth, and your baby, and you
are entitled to all the power that those facts provide.

This book will give you everything you need to know so you won't be left wondering what could have been. Knowing what birthing options there are will allow you to make informed choices and have an empowered childbirth experience. I will share my personal experiences and nuggets of wisdom through unfiltered tips and suggestions that will inform and guide you on your childbearing journey. I'll cover everything pregnancy: handling the highs and lows of the journey; figuring out your birth preferences and the place that's right for you; and knowing all your options. Then I'll go over laboring and birthing tips and scenarios, and how to deal with everything going right or wrong. Finally, I'll talk about the often neglected fourth trimester: self-care, infant care, being cared for, and so much more. I am not scared to talk about everything—the real deal, unfiltered birth in all its beautiful and messy glory—and I want to make sure you aren't scared either.

Lindsey Bliss

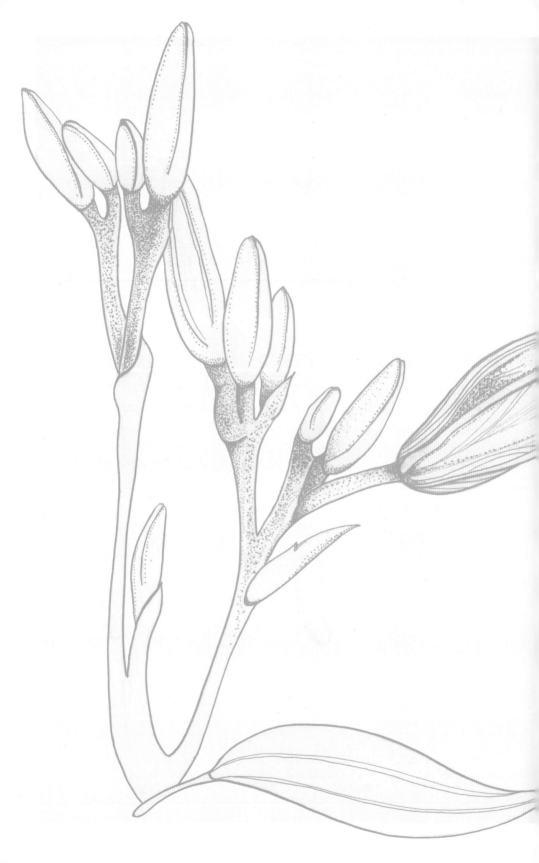

Part One
Your Pregnancy

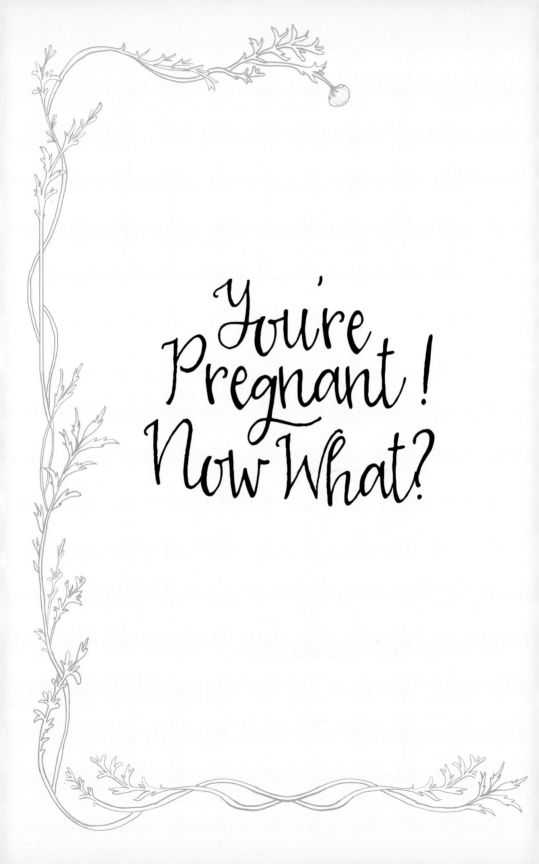

You're Pregnant! Now What?

YOUR PATH TO BECOMING PREGNANT MAY HAVE BEEN meticulously planned, or it may have been a complete surprise. You may have needed assistance in becoming pregnant, or your birth control may have failed. You may be having a rainbow baby after an infant loss or miscarriage. No matter what the road has been like, take a big, deep breath and honor your journey to becoming pregnant. All our stories are wonderfully different. Be open to processing any feelings and emotions that may come up when you find out that you are pregnant. Excitement may not be your first and only emotional response, and that's okay. There is no manual or rulebook on how to feel or how to process this life-altering news. Be gentle on yourself. The range of possible responses is vast and varied. News of a pregnancy can be dark and scary; not everyone celebrates it. I processed through shock, fear, grief, and awe before I even got close to excitement. I had one doula client tell me that she was in such an extreme state of shock that she didn't make an official pregnancy announcement until her final weeks of pregnancy. Another client was so overcome with joy that she literally wet her pants from the uncontrollable glee giggles!

You may pee on four or five pregnancy tests before the news really sinks in. Well, I did, anyway. I tried every single brand and type of home urine pregnancy test, because I know they are not always accurate for every person. Some people get negative pregnancy test results but are indeed pregnant. My aunt, for example, never had a positive urine pregnancy test and only confirmed her pregnancy through a missed period and a blood test. She also got a baby at the end—how's that for confirmation?!

ESTIMATING YOUR DUE DATE

You're *pregnant*! Now what? First, figure out your estimated due date. Did you notice that I used the word *estimated*? Even if you know exactly when you conceived, and even if you had fertility assistance, you can't be completely certain as to when your little one will be joining you

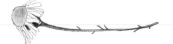

earth-side. There is no due-date crystal ball, especially at this early stage of the game. I like to refer to a "due month" instead of a "due date."

Our ancestors used the phases of the moon to predict when babies would be born. An average menstruation cycle is twenty-eight days, and the moon has a similar cycle. This method proved to be very accurate. Even today, many care providers and birth workers swear that the full moon brings all the babies. This has not been scientifically proven, but the thinking is: When the moon is full, its gravitational pull creates high tides, and because we are made up of mostly water, this can throw us into labor. I'd like to believe that we are all in sync with the powerful energy of the moon, and I'm going to guard that belief. My husband is a surfer, and he *always* accurately predicts when my clients will go into labor based on the waves that day.

Today, most care providers count forty weeks from the first day of your last menstrual cycle to estimate your due date. Please remember that a normal pregnancy ranges from thirty-eight to forty-two weeks. That's a five-week span of when you may give birth, and only 5 percent of people deliver on their actual due date. Out of all my births, only my last baby came right on her due date. I'm proof that it's not impossible, but it's not very likely either. Try surrendering to the process and trusting that your baby knows when to come.

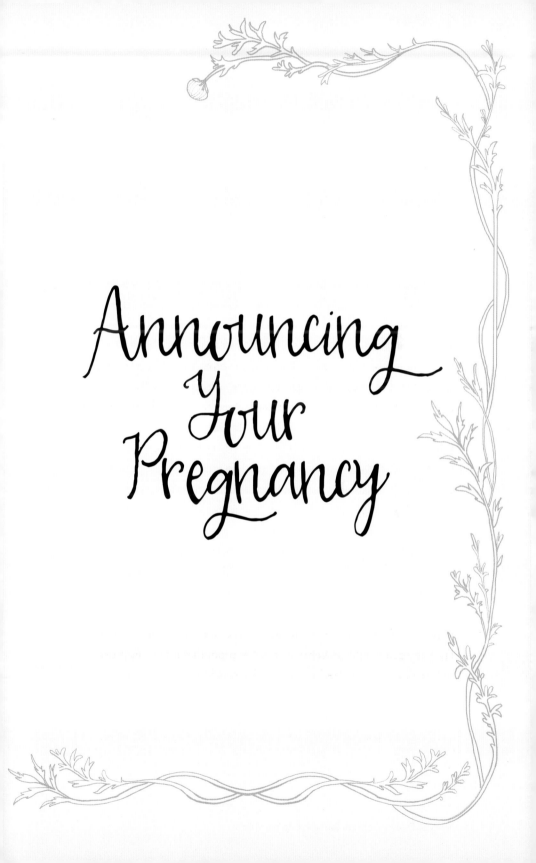

Announcing Your Pregnancy

ONCE YOUR PREGNANCY HAS BEEN CONFIRMED BY A missed period or a positive pregnancy test and you have an idea of what your due date is, you may feel like your prayers have been answered, or you may be coming out of a heavy fog of denial and shock. Depending on your circumstances, sharing the news of your pregnancy may be extremely exciting or filled with anxiety.

In today's culture, many people announce their pregnancy to friends and family via social media. You can go that route, or you can make your big announcement in person at a family gathering or holiday event. I often announced my pregnancies by simply making good old-fashioned phone calls. I vividly remember the life-altering phone call I made to tell my husband that we were having twins. He had skipped the ultrasound appointment during which I found out, and he didn't believe me at first. Then followed a tidal wave of shock. Why the hell would I make that one up? Fast-forward to my next pregnancy: We went a bit grander and announced our second twin pregnancy (yes, *second*!) at a family gathering. I figured I would show them my growing bump to make sure that they *really* believed me.

Many folks wait until around twelve to fourteen weeks into the pregnancy to announce it. This marks the start of your second trimester and a point in your pregnancy at which the risk of miscarriage drastically drops. Perhaps you are pregnant with your rainbow baby and you would prefer not to announce your pregnancy until the third trimester; that's absolutely fine, too. It's your announcement, and you should make it whenever and in whatever way feels comfortable to you.

According to the American Congress of Obstetricians and Gynecologists (ACOG), 10 to 25 percent of all pregnancies end in miscarriage. It is beneficial to have some knowledge about miscarriage in the unfortunate event that it happens to you or someone you know. There is a lot of silence and misinformation surrounding it. It's a club no one wants to join, but once you're in it, you may find out that many people you know have experienced a miscarriage too. You are *not* alone.

on Miscarriages and Rainbow Babies

by Jessica Zucker, Ph.D., *Psychologist and Founder of the*
#IHadAMiscarriage Campaign

A rainbow baby is a baby that follows a miscarriage, pregnancy loss, stillbirth, neonatal death, or infant loss. The name comes from that the fact that, environmentally, rainbows often follow storms, inspiring hope for calmer days. The storm symbolizes the pregnancy loss, while the rainbow represents the baby that follows. It behooves us culturally and personally to discuss rainbow mamas and rainbow babies in part because of the anxiety and fear often associated with pregnancy after pregnancy loss. The trauma of loss reverberates, and countless women walk on eggshells through subsequent pregnancies, terrified that loss may occur again. Furthermore, even once the rainbow baby arrives, some women report experiencing anxiety about the baby's continued survival. Anecdotally, women who have rainbow babies share having different relationships—emotionally speaking—with their rainbow baby versus other children. Loss can have resounding effects on women and their families. Grief is as individual as pregnancy.

Tons of places offer support after pregnancy loss. Here are some resources I find valuable:

Pregnancy After Loss Support: www.pregnancyafterlosssupport.com
Miscarriage Association: www.miscarriageassociation.org.uk
Organizations that Provide Support after Miscarriage/Stillbirth/ Infant Loss:
www.verywell.com/miscarriage-support-organizations-2371339
#IHadAMiscarriage Campaign: www.instagram.com/ihadamiscarriage

There are many local and online resources for miscarriage support. Keeping the lines of communication open with family, friends, and care providers can also help you get the support you need to process this tremendous loss. It's okay to not be okay.

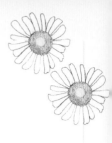

MY FIRST BIRTH

Mia Josephine
March 10, 2006
Hospital Birthing Center

This is the birth story of my firstborn, Mia. She was my first pregnancy, my first childbirth, and my first baby. I did have a little bit of experience with kids because of my stepdaughter, Bella, whom I met when she was eight. I adore Bella, and I was really looking forward to giving her a little baby sister. Bella was a great and easy kid, so I really had no idea what I was in for with a baby. When Dan (my now-husband) and I first started to get serious, we had "the baby talk." He was content just having his daughter and had no desire to have any more kids. I agreed that I wasn't ready at the time, but I needed to be in a relationship in which kids could be a possibility in the future. I was in my early twenties and knew I might change my mind. He agreed, saying that we would cross that bridge when and if we came to it. Little did I know that we would be crossing it very soon.

My close friend had recently told me that she was pregnant. I couldn't believe it. Most of our friends were still caught up in partying and being irresponsible. I realized that I didn't remember when my last period was. My friend was convinced that I was pregnant too. She was actually hoping I was. I took a pregnancy test, and it was negative. I was relieved, because I didn't feel ready. Do you ever? At the time, I didn't know it was possible to have a false negative pregnancy test. I took two more tests over the next few weeks, and the third one came out positive. I was shocked. At the time, I might have been the least likely person on the planet to have a baby. The majority of my friends agreed. I walked around in a daze for the first few months just trying to digest the news. Then I started to get excited.

I knew from the beginning that I wanted an unmedicated birth. I had read Ina May Gaskin's book *Spiritual Midwifery* when I was a teenager, mostly because it had cool pictures of long-haired naked folks.

My mother was a Bradley childbirth instructor when I was a kid, so she always had birthing books lying around our house. It was natural curiosity, I guess.

I found a birthing center and hired a birth doula. My birth doula had given birth to a bunch of kids herself, and she reminded me of a fertility goddess. She had a calming energy that I appreciated. My pregnancy was uncomplicated and relatively easy. I did, however, gain almost 75 pounds (34 kg). I was a little underweight when I got pregnant, and my pregnant best friend liked to feed me root beer floats. It was nice to have a pregnancy buddy: We spent lots of time discussing every detail of our pregnancies and our birth plans. We used the same midwifery practice and chose the same birthing center. She delivered her daughter four days before I did in the same exact room. It was beautifully serendipitous, or at least it ended up that way after quite a ride.

I was forty weeks and one day pregnant when I decided to self-induce with castor oil. (Disclaimer: Do not do this!) I made this decision impulsively and regret that I didn't wait for labor to start on its own. I took way too much and did not consult my midwife or birth doula. I went to bed that night thinking that the castor oil wasn't going to work. Then I woke up around 3 a.m. with strong contractions two to three minutes apart. I called my doula and midwife and headed to the birthing center. I threw up, with my head out of the car window, the entire ride to the hospital. When my husband and I arrived, we couldn't find the entrance. I labored on my hands and knees outside on the sidewalk. It must have been a pretty funny sight. I wasn't laughing. After what felt like an eternity, we eventually found the hospital entrance.

When they checked me in, I was only 4 cm dilated. The midwives wanted me to be dilated closer to 5 or 6 cm before admitting me to the birthing center. But while in the triage area, I dropped to my knees, moaning. The nurses took pity on me and agreed to admit me just in case my labor was progressing quickly. I'm so glad they did. I hopped in the tub around the same time my birth doula arrived. She had a calming presence, and I was glad that she was there. I was moaning and howling loudly throughout the entire laboring process. I didn't want anyone to touch me, and I felt very out of control. I never really got a break between contractions. I got out of the tub after a short period of time and got on the bed. I started to get the urge to bear down. They checked me and I was fully dilated. I went from 4 cm to 10 cm dilated in one hour! They were all shocked. I didn't even really push, either. My baby was like a Mack truck coming out: fast and furious. I really thought my legs were going to snap off my body. She came out so fast that her cord snapped in half. It turned out her cord was much shorter than a normal umbilical cord. I hemorrhaged a bit, and they had to check me for retained placenta. That part was really painful.

The birth was very fast and felt out of control. I think the castor oil may have played a part in that; it may have greased the pipes a little too much. I did, however, get the natural birth I had wanted. It went so quickly that I couldn't even think to ask for pain management. It really helped to be in a birthing center that supported my desire for an unmedicated birth. It was one of the most painful, scary, and beautiful experiences of my entire life. I'll never forget seeing Mia's little face and sweet eyes for the first time.

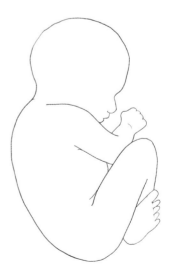

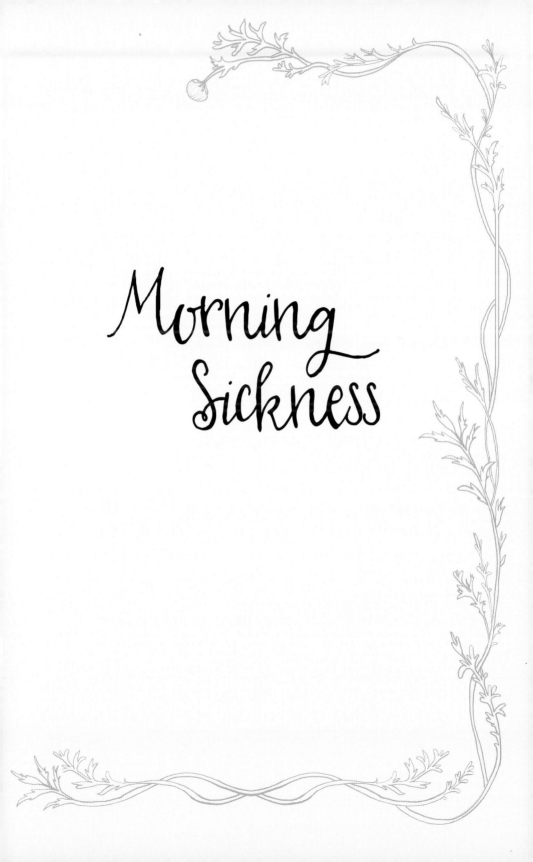

Morning Sickness

MORNING SICKNESS, AKA NAUSEA GRAVIDARUM, AFFECTS 80 percent of all pregnant people. You may get nauseous, vomit, and/ or feel absolutely exhausted. It's called *morning sickness* because some people feel sick in the morning and gradually feel better as the day progresses. For other not-so-lucky folks, it can last all damn day!

The symptoms vary from person to person. I personally felt severely hungover (minus the drinking, obviously) every morning for about four months. Why does this happen? Doctors think it's caused by your body's reaction to the significant increase of hormones during the first trimester, but they aren't entirely certain. Nausea can begin as early as your fourth week of pregnancy and commonly ends around your fourteenth week. Some folks stay sick for the entire pregnancy. I'm sending good vibes and crossing my fingers that this won't happen to you!

Severe morning sickness is called *hyperemesis gravidarum*. It can be so bad that you may vomit multiple times a day, become dehydrated, and/or lose weight instead of gaining it. You might even need to visit the doctor to receive intravenous rehydration. The chances of this super-intense bout of morning sickness are heightened when you are pregnant with multiples, if you're prone to migraines, or if you have a history of motion sickness. I scored a 3 out of 3 on this list! I also know a fellow twin mother who had such a bad case of hyperemesis gravidrum

---

EXPERT TIP

on Morning Sickness

by Robin Rose Bennett, *Writer, Green Witch, Herbalist, Wisewoman, and Founder of Wisewoman Healing Ways*

Slow, steady sipping of ginger tea, especially made from freshly grated root, is quite effective for many women. I also like ginger powder rolled into balls with raw, local honey as an alternative. They are easy to carry with you in a little tin.

on Morning Sickness

by Miracle Mattie, *My Grandmother, Herbalist, and Massage Therapist*

Drink this fresh ginger tea daily, first thing upon waking, to battle morning sickness.

1–2-inch (2.5–5 cm) piece fresh ginger root, peeled and grated
1 teaspoon raw honey, or to taste, optional
Squeeze lemon juice, or to taste, optional

Bring ginger and 2 cups (470 ml) water to a boil in a small, covered pot. Boil for 5 minutes. Strain, pour into a mug, and add honey and lemon. Serve immediately.

(vomiting fifteen times or more a day!) that she was hospitalized three times for severe dehydration. She then needed Zofran, a medication for extreme nausea that's administered through a peripherally inserted central catheter (PICC) line. She lost 15 pounds (7 kg) in the first two trimesters of pregnancy. This is obviously an extreme case, but know that you are not alone if you suffer from hyperemesis gravidrum during your pregnancy.

Here are a few ways that you can try to find relief from your morning sickness. It doesn't hurt to ask your care provider for tips too.

Eating small, frequent meals can help. I felt like a squirrel getting ready for winter by storing small snacks in every pocket or bag that I carried. I always kept almonds on my nightstand to battle my morning and late-night stomach upset. Protein seemed to really help. I also used peppermint essential oil when a wave of nausea hit. I'd dab a bit on my wrists and temples, and it really helped to soothe my stomach. I've also heard that lemon oil can do the trick. I would highly recommend getting an essential oil diffuser for your home. It was a game changer for me. I drank most of my water with a lemon wedge, and just the smell of a freshly cut lemon would settle my stomach. There have been a few studies suggesting that vitamin B_6 supplements can also do the trick. Doctors aren't sure why this works, but it does seem to help.

My daily fifteen-minute pregnancy meditation practice of deep belly breathing was another thing that really helped quell my nausea. I would focus on my inhales and exhales while feeling my belly rise and fall. I would also repeat in my head the mantra, "This will not last forever," or "I am growing a baby." You are breathing for two beings. One of my doula clients liked the mantra, "This is only a baby-growing hangover." This simple practice was extremely helpful in keeping me feeling good during a few of my challenging puke-filled pregnancies.

I felt like a squirrel getting ready for winter by storing small snacks in every pocket or bag that I carried.

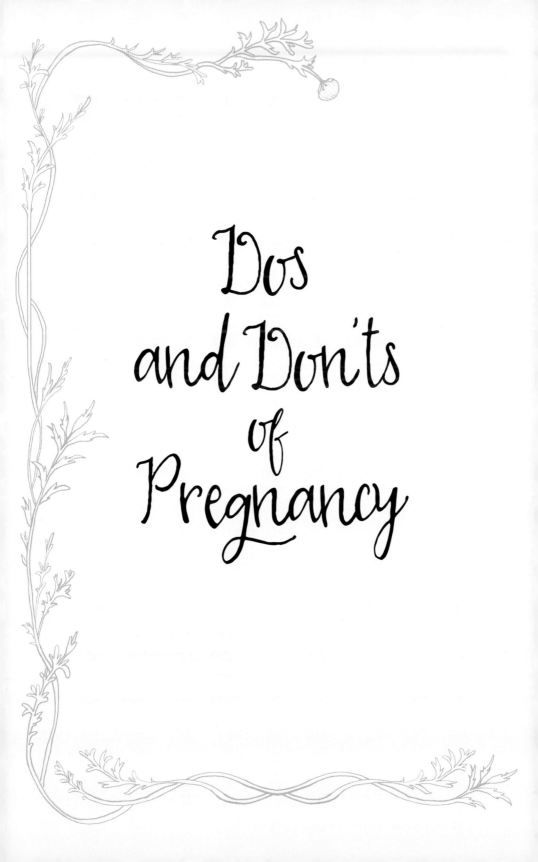

Dos
and Don'ts
of
Pregnancy

NOW THAT YOU'RE PREGNANT, I'M SURE YOU'RE WONDER-ing about the dos and don'ts of pregnancy. I hear a lot of different pregnancy-related concerns from my doula clients that often lead to too much internet searching and unnecessary stress and fear. Some things are worth worrying about, and others are not. Here is a simple guide to help you navigate the start of your childbearing journey.

DO LIST

Do find a care provider that you like and trust. Yes, liking your care provider is just as important as trusting your care provider. You will feel much more comfortable asking all the pregnancy- and childbirth-related questions that pop up. Please, please, please like your care provider.

Do surround yourself with supportive and positive people. If you have any toxic relationships in your life, now is the best time to step away from them. It's not worth the stress on you and your growing baby. Surround yourself with a force field of love.

Do your research. If you don't know what your choices are, you don't have any. Watch a few birth documentaries, read the books, and take a tour of your local birthing facilities. Knowledge is power. Consider hiring a doula to help you navigate your childbearing journey. A doula is a person who is trained to assist you during childbirth. If you cannot afford a doula, try contacting a local doula collective anyway, because they may have doulas-in-training whose services are low cost or even free. Many new doulas will volunteer their services to gain experience. I always try to make room in my personal doula practice to offer a sliding scale fee or pro bono work. You deserve support if you want it. (For more information on the role of a doula, see page 68.)

Do trust your intuition. It never leads you astray; it only looks to guide you. Listen to your gut.

Do exercise. If you are healthy and not having a high-risk pregnancy, exercise is just fine. Please review your exercise of choice with your care provider to make sure it's right for you at this moment. It's definitely not the time to learn how to do handstands or take up tightrope walking if you haven't already mastered these skills prior to pregnancy.

Do have sex. Go ahead and get freaky. Unless you are deemed high risk by your care provider, sex is considered safe throughout your entire pregnancy. Your amniotic sac and the muscles of the uterus help to protect your baby. Be mindful, though, that sex can sometimes cause some mild contractions or cramping. Also, don't feel bad if you are *not* in the mood and don't want to have sex at all. Your libido may disappear. Honor however you are feeling.

Do eat well. Your vessel is sacred. Treat it that way by putting the best food into it. You and your baby deserve it. If possible, cut out most, if not all, sugar. Eat real food. You are not *really* supposed to be eating for two. Yes, you will need more calories, but only a few hundred more. Try 300 to 500 extra calories. I live my life following the 80/20 rule: For 80 percent of the time, I eat super-duper well. For 20 percent of the time, I indulge myself with a vanilla ice cream sandwich, raw chocolate, or a cupcake with rainbow sprinkles. Yes, I have a wicked sweet tooth.

> *Fact:*
> Sugar is far more addictive than cocaine.

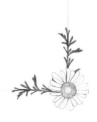

Do rest. You are growing a freakin' human being. Your body is doing major work. This can be physically and emotionally exhausting. Rest as much as you can. If you can sleep in, *do it*!

Do hydrate. You need more water than usual now that you are pregnant—like twelve to thirteen 8-ounce (235 ml) glasses a day! Keeping hydrated prevents constipation. I hate not being regular, so that was enough for me to remember to drink enough water. Your skin also benefits from your hydrating efforts as well. Bonus!

Do meditate. Meditation helps clear the static in your brain. How can you listen to your intuition if you can't even collect your thoughts? Anxiety and fear cloud your inner voice. Practicing meditation will help bring clarity to your decision making. This will help you navigate your pregnancy with mindfulness.

DON'T LIST

Don't rely on Dr. Google for answers. Falling down the internet research rabbit hole can cause lots of unnecessary anxiety and many misdiagnosed conditions.

Don't hang around folks who only want to tell you their birth horror stories. I'm not entirely sure what compels people to try and scare the living daylights out of you, but please realize that most of these stories are not the norm. None of these stories helped me with *any* of my births. What they did do was contribute to my high levels of anxiety and made me fear childbirth. Tell them to share their horror stories with you *after* your baby is born.

Don't be bullied into any decision based on fear. Educate yourself about your options and find a care provider that practices evidence-based care (see page 75). Every care provider has a different recipe for childbirth. You are the consumer, and you get to decide which one is right for you.

Don't smoke. I mean, really? Do I have to tell you why this is harmful to you and your baby? Well, I will. Smoking *doubles* the risk of a stillbirth. Talk to your physician about quitting if you are currently a smoker.

Don't clean the kitty litter box. You deserve a break from it anyway! In addition, there is a risk of toxoplasmosis, a parasitic infection contracted by cleaning the litter box of an infected cat. Gross, right? It's also dangerous for your unborn child. If you don't have someone to clean the kitty box for you, please wear protective gloves.

Don't drink too much caffeine. One cup of coffee a day is fine; just don't overdo it. Thank the heavens for that one cup a day, though. When I was pregnant with my second set of twins, I *needed* my morning cup of joe just to get my engine running. Skip the soda, though. That crap rots out your teeth and is filled with that devil, sugar.

Don't stress. The way you live your life is the way you will birth your baby. A stress-filled pregnancy is often followed by a stressful childbirth experience. Surrender to the flow of things. Trust the process. Even the darkest of days and experiences will have a silver lining.

Don't eat unsafe food. Unpasteurized milk and cheeses may contain bacteria such as *E. coli*, *Listeria*, or *Salmonella*. FoodSafety.gov, which is run by the U.S. Department of Health and Human Services, says to steer clear of sushi due to potential risk of parasites or bacteria, but I have a confession to make: I ate sushi during all my pregnancies. I skipped the tuna and the oily fish due to their increased mercury levels, and I always bought my sushi from a very high-quality restaurant and never from somewhere like a gas station rest stop. My kids turned out just fine. You should talk to your care provider to get a full list of the foods to avoid and talk over any exceptions you might want to make.

Don't drink booze. The ACOG advises abstaining from all alcohol while pregnant. In American culture, we tend to be overindulgent by nature and enjoy things in excess. I'm pretty sure that's why the majority of care providers in the United States say no to all alcohol consumption while pregnant. Some less conservative obstetricians and midwives have said that a small glass of wine occasionally won't hurt your growing babe, and there are some recent studies in the UK that support this. I have never only wanted a small glass of wine in my entire life. A few sips for me always lead to a very full glass of wine and then maybe a second. So I opted to just skip the drinking while pregnant, as skipping booze poses no risks to the baby.

Don't skip the childbirth education class. Some folks just like to wing it, but I would strongly caution against that. There is tremendous value in attending these lessons. Educating yourself on all the things that can potentially unfold during your birth will prepare you for all possibilities. You will also learn about what your birthing options are in the city or town where you are giving birth. If you don't like the group setting, consider a private or an online class. Look for one that supports your birthing philosophies.

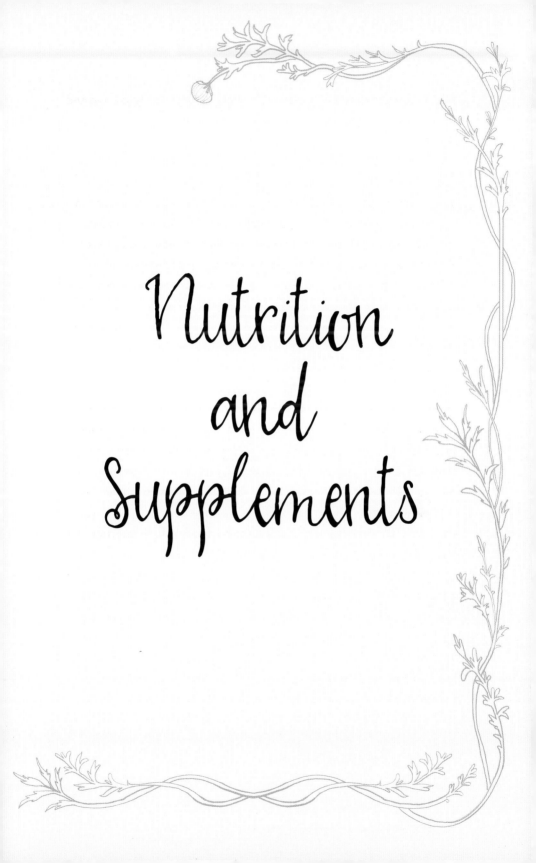

Nutrition and Supplements

THE FOOD THAT YOU PUT INTO YOUR BODY IS FUEL, AND during pregnancy it is important to fill up your tank with premium quality fuel. The digested nutrients will pass through the umbilical cord and into the baby's bloodstream. Most people start their pregnancy depleted of many nutrients, so care providers typically suggest taking a prenatal supplement to replenish your stores. I have found that prenatal whole food supplements are the easiest on the stomach. Whole food supplements are made from concentrated extracts of whole foods. They have lower levels of iron and folic acid, nutrients that tend to cause stomach irritability. This will be especially important if you are experiencing morning sickness. The conventional prenatal vitamins also made me very constipated, which was yet another reason I opted for whole food supplements. The downside is that they are more expensive. For me, the additional cost was well worth it.

Another supplement that may be suggested during pregnancy is iron, which plays an important role in the production of blood and circulating the oxygen in blood around the body. Your blood volume increases by 50 percent during pregnancy, so iron is a key nutrient. Anemia, most commonly caused by an iron deficiency, is a condition in which you lack enough red blood cells to carry oxygen throughout your body, and it can lead to extreme fatigue and weakness. Anemia can also be caused by vitamin B_{12} and folate deficiencies. Risks associated with anemia include preterm labor and postpartum hemorrhage. I was slightly anemic during both of my twin pregnancies, and I later learned that twin pregnancies can increase your chances of becoming anemic. I would suggest finding a non-constipating liquid iron supplement that is easier on your stomach. Please discuss this and all your prenatal vitamin options with your care provider.

Next, *eat real food*! You don't need to see a nutritionist to know that eating processed food is not good for you or your growing baby. Processed foods and fast foods can contain genetically modified grains and genetically engineered ingredients. Their negative effects are still unknown, and they should be avoided. Eat organic and local foods

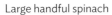

Green Smoothie

Large handful spinach
1 cup (235 ml) almond milk, plus more for blending if necessary
1 large tablespoon (16 g) almond butter
1 banana

Blend on high speed in a blender, adding more almond milk if necessary, until smoothie reaches desired consistency. Serve immediately.

whenever possible. I know that this can be quite costly, so just do the best you can. I loved frequenting my local farmer's market every week during pregnancy to stock up on all my favorite leafy green vegetables.

According to the World Health Organization, a healthy diet during pregnancy contains adequate protein, vitamins, and minerals obtained through the consumption of a variety of foods, including green and orange vegetables, meat, fish, beans, nuts, pasteurized dairy products, and fruit.

I'm sure you have heard, but refined sugar is the devil. Really. It is. Greatly reducing your sugar intake will decrease your risk of gestational diabetes and other pregnancy complications. Don't fret, fruit is fine to eat in moderation. Whole fruits only contain a small amount of fructose, and the benefits of fruit outweigh the risks.

PREGNANCY SUPERFOODS

Including a few of these pregnancy superfoods in your diet can ensure that you and your growing babe are getting enough nutrients.

Avocados are jam-packed with nutrients and healthy fats. I cut one in half for breakfast and dig in with a spoon. Easy peasy! Avocados are high in potassium, which can help ease those middle-of-the-night charley

SOUL FOOD RITUAL BATH

by Deborah Hanekamp, aka Mama Medicine, seeress in the
healing arts as an initiated Amazonian shaman, reiki master,
and yogini

When body, mind, and spirit are in need of nourishment, I like to take
this bath while listening to Billie Holiday and sipping nettle tea.

Ingredients

1 cup (270 g) salt

1 tablespoon (15 ml) apple cider vinegar

A few drops sweet orange essential oil

1 candle (I like white, unscented candles)

1 cinnamon stick

Amethyst and black tourmaline crystals

1 mug tea brewed with ½ teaspoon calendula, ½ teaspoon nettles, and a
    pinch nori

A relaxing, healing book such as *The Gift* by Hafiz

Ritual

- Draw a warm bath and add the salt, vinegar, and sweet orange essential oil to the water.

- Light your candle.

- From the flame, bless yourself with the smoke of a cinnamon stick.

- Step into the bath, and dunk your head under water.

- Infuse the water with a prayer that you feel is nurturing of health and well-being.

- Hold the amethyst to your third eye, then your heart, and then anywhere you need restorative energy.

- Practice Nadi Shodhana* breathing.

- Sip your tea, and read your book.

- When you are ready to end your bath, press your hands to your heart in gratitude.

* Nadi Shodhana is alternate nostril breathing. In Sanskrit, *nadii* means "flow" and *shodhana* means "purification." In practicing Nadi Shodhana, you are clearing the channels of the mind and body. Focus on inhaling through the left nostril, and exhaling through the right nostril. Then inhale through the left nostril and exhale through the right. Repeat.

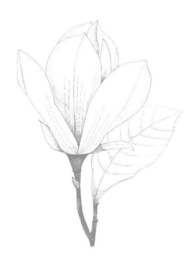

on Protein

by Jessica Prescott, *author of* Vegan Goodness *and Founder of the Blog* Wholy Goodness

If you're craving sweets, you need more protein, something I wish I knew sooner because I had a seeeeerious sweet tooth during pregnancy. I ate a lot of protein in the form of peanut butter, beans, lentils, nuts, and veggies, but I also ate a lot of vegan chocolate and cake. Make a black bean brownie or banana–peanut butter smoothie and get your protein and sweet fix in one hit.

horses. One of my doula clients was absolutely obsessed with making guacamole every day for breakfast! There really is nothing quite as healthy or delicious as homemade guacamole. These are the good fats.

According to a study published in 2011 in the *Journal of Obstetrics and Gynaecology*, dates are said to strengthen your amniotic sac to help prevent premature rupture of membranes, increase your chances of spontaneous labor, and reduce your overall time in labor. The study suggests consuming six dates a day for the four weeks leading up to your due date. Dates have much more sugar than you realize, so I'd recommend consuming a couple instead of six. Try adding a few dates to a smoothie every so often or eat one as a treat, but consume in moderation. Dates are great, but don't overdo it on the sugar.

Leafy greens ruled my pregnancy world. I loved eating sautéed spinach or a kale salad, and I craved them as much as ice cream. Hard to believe, right? But spinach smoothies are my favorite. I made one *every* morning during my last pregnancy. Greens are high in fiber and rich in folate. Win-win.

on Taking Iron

by Jessica Prescott, *author of* Vegan Goodness *and Founder of the Blog* Wholy Goodness

One of the things that confused me most during pregnancy was when to take my iron. Take it on an empty stomach, they say. Two hours before eating food, they say. Ummmm, when is a pregnant woman ever not grazing? Seriously. My solution to this was to take it right before I went to bed, or during one of my many nighttime trips to the bathroom.

My obsession, during pregnancy and through to today, is eating sauerkraut and kimchi. Fermented foods are rich with probiotic (good) bacteria, which are linked with improving your gut health and boosting immunity in you and your baby.

Remember the 80/20 rule. If you eat well most of the time, you can enjoy that ice cream sundae, guilt free!

DRINK SO MUCH WATER

Hydrate. Hydrate. Hydrate. I would highly suggest purchasing a flashy, neon-colored water bottle so that it pretty much shouts at you to take a sip whenever you look at. I personally find it harder to forget it at home or to lose a water bottle when it's a bright, obnoxious color.

If you become dehydrated during your pregnancy, you will have issues with overheating. This is typically why pregnant folks are always boiling hot. They're dehydrated! On the other hand, being well hydrated can help prevent hemorrhoids, headaches, nausea, constipation, and

on Hydration

by Jessica Prescott, *author of* Vegan Goodness *and Founder of the Blog* Wholy Goodness

Every time you feel like putting something in your mouth, drink a glass of water first. You'll be surprised at how often that desire to eat was a misinterpreted cue from your body that you need to hydrate yourself.

tiredness. Be mindful that in the last months of your pregnancy, being dehydrated can lead to premature labor. When you're dehydrated, your blood volume decreases and oxytocin increases, which can trigger contractions. Check your pee to make sure it's a nice clear color and not dark yellow.

Eat real food! Eating processed food is not good for you or your growing baby.

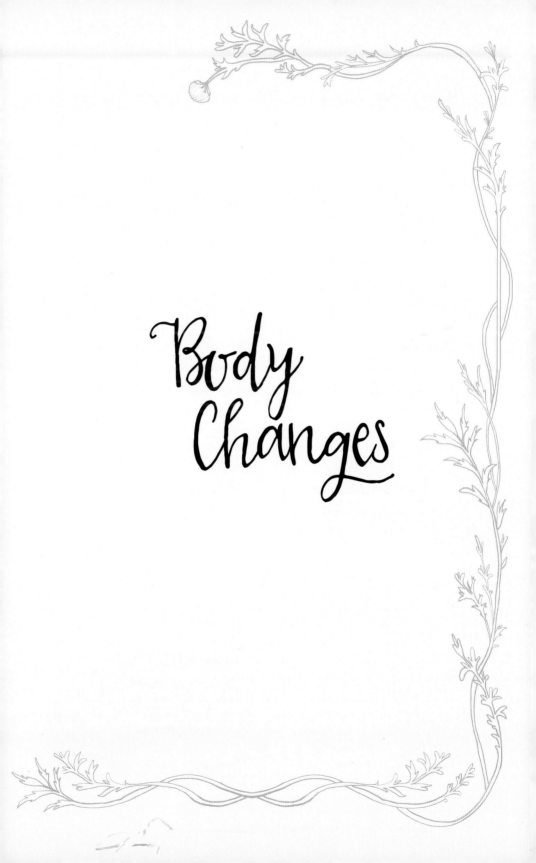

Body
Changes

COMING TO TERMS WITH YOUR RAPIDLY CHANGING PREG-
nant body can be extremely challenging. During my pregnancies, lots of
the physical changes that unfolded left me wondering, "Is this normal?"
Our current culture is so obsessed with appearances that we rarely even
hear about body changes that can occur during pregnancy. I'd love your
help in creating a body-positive culture that embraces these changes and
even celebrates our changing bodies because we are growing and carrying a new life. If celebrating these changes doesn't feel right to you—and
no one will blame you if it doesn't, as they can be challenging and even
painful—at least this chapter can help you become well informed and
prepared.

STRETCH MARKS

Everywhere you look, there is an advertisement for a stretch mark cream.
Just the other day, I was watching television and a commercial for a
celebrity-endorsed miracle stretch mark cream popped up. Through
this deluge in the media, we are being taught that we must avoid stretch
marks at all costs. I'd like to know why. I ended up with some on my
breasts, bum, thighs, and belly, and they are all physical proof of what my

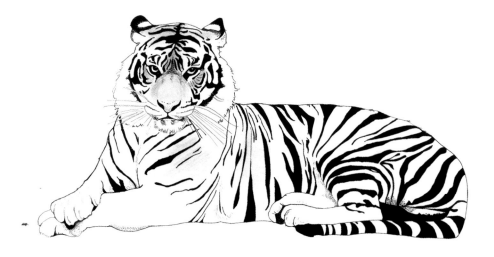

Piercings and Stretch Marks

If you have, or had, a belly button piercing, there is a very high likelihood that a stretch mark will appear at that spot. The area around the ring may become irritated and prone to infection. With proper hygiene, you can leave it in, but it may become uncomfortable.

body is capable of. I am damn proud of my warrior-mama tiger stripes! Believe it or not, I love them.

Listen, folks, you either get them or you don't. It's genetics. No magic balm will steer you completely clear of stretch marks or erase them once you have them. I'd recommend saving your money on magic creams and just buying some coconut oil. It will nourish, moisturize, sooth, and heal your stretching skin. Rub it everywhere. I recommend applying coconut oil to your body every night before you hit the hay. Many of my doula clients who are expecting twins end up with stretch marks. I always remind them of the fact that they are stretching to accommodate not one but *two* babies. What a magnificent feat!

VEINS

Veins, stretch marks, and cellulite. Oh my! Why didn't anyone tell me that I could get a varicose vein on my labia? When I was on my second pregnancy, which was with twins, I looked like I was smuggling a Twinkie on only one side of my underwear. As your uterus grows during pregnancy, it puts added pressure on the inferior vena cava (the large vein on the right side of your body), which in turn puts pressure on veins in the leg and/or pelvic region, and varicose veins can pop out in that whole area. Exercise and good nutrition can help prevent varicose veins, but genetics also play a role. Thanks, Mom! And although varicose veins don't always hurt, the one on my labium sure did. Wearing compression

on Varicose Veins

by Robin Rose Bennett, *writer, green witch, herbalist, wisewoman, and founder of Wisewoman Healing Ways*

Increase circulation safely with tasty grape leaf or nettle leaf infusion. Pour boiling water over about 1 cup (70 g) of herbs per quart (1 L) glass jar and steep them, covered and as airtight as possible, for about 8 hours. Then squeeze the herbs into the infusion to gain the maximum potency and compost the leaves. This can be refrigerated and reheated for use or heated and stored in a stainless steel thermos. You can also wash the legs with a washcloth dipped into either of these teas.

tights saved my life. Thank you, Spanx! My hope is that you will avoid vulvar varicosities altogether, but if you don't, just know that you are *not* alone. Many of my clients claim to have found relief from varicose veins by maintaining a regular prenatal yoga practice. Prenatal yoga is also a great choice for exercise during your pregnancy. It's win-win!

Next up, spider veins. Spider veins are small, thin, blue or red blood vessels that can be seen under the skin. They appear in a pattern similar to a spider web or sunburst. It is more common to have these pesky veins appear and/or get more severe in an additional pregnancy after the first one. They pop up most commonly on the legs or the face. Spider veins are typically more unsightly than they are uncomfortable. They can sometimes, however, feel itchy or even crampy. Thankfully, they are usually only a temporary side effect of pregnancy and often go away post-delivery, so don't worry about them if you do get them. My late grandmother's home remedy for spider veins was to apply witch hazel with a cotton ball a few times a day until they went away. The astringent properties help cure the veins. She swore by it. To lessen the risk of getting spider veins, try not to stand for too long, put your feet up often, and try not to cross your legs while sitting.

ACNE

That radiant pregnancy glow can sometimes be accompanied by a bad case of acne. You can blame it on the hormone (progesterone) surges and perhaps that extra helping of ice cream. Your body is retaining fluids, which contain toxins that result in pimples. These pimples don't just pop up on your face either; some of us are lucky enough to get them all over our rear ends. Fun, right? I suggest hydrating, and perhaps skipping the ice cream, to help clear up your skin if you're experiencing outbreaks.

I don't recommend using your normal face wash or acne treatments. Tons of beauty products contain ingredients you absolutely don't want to absorb while pregnant. You can find out about chemical-free skin cleansers on the website of the Environmental Working Group (EWG), a well-known organization that rates products according to their ingredients. They'll even tell you what specific health concerns are caused by a particular ingredient. I suggest always checking with your care provider, too, if you are unsure of any ingredients in a product you want to use.

I had one doula client claim that she was allergic to being pregnant with boys. During her first pregnancy with her daughter, she had radiant, glowing skin. During her second pregnancy with her son, however, her skin broke out like she was a teenager with a pizza face. I'm pretty sure that there is no scientific research to back her claim, but she certainly believes it!

CONSTIPATION

Oh poop! We can blame pregnancy hormones for constipation, too, because they relax and slow down the bowels. Your growing uterus is also taking up space, making it harder for your bowels to do their job. To keep things moving as best they can, hydrate, hydrate, hydrate, and eat fiber-rich foods. The more spinach and watermelon that I consumed during pregnancy, the more I pooped. Watermelon juice has been my #1 cure for pregnancy constipation.

on Constipation

by Robin Rose Bennett, *writer, green witch, herbalist, wisewoman, and founder of Wisewoman Healing Ways*

Keep slippery elm powder on hand in your kitchen "pharmacy." My favorite approach to constipation is to peel and then cut up a red (or yellow or green) apple, preferably organic. Cook it in a little water, just enough to cover the apple, 15–20 minutes, until soft. Stir in ground cinnamon to taste and 1 teaspoon slippery elm powder. Additionally, daily use of 1 spoonful or more of slippery elm in whole-fat plain yogurt is an excellent preventive remedy.

EXPERT TIP

on Constipation Relief

by Tara Stiles, *yoga instructor and founder of Strala Yoga*

Oh constipation! One of the fun and surprising features of pregnancy. A consistent, easygoing yoga practice can go a long way toward keeping all things regular. Allowing the mind to release and relax signals the body to follow. Plus, moving around a bit with standing and balancing poses will also get your energy up. Give yourself extra time and take extra big breaths when releasing moves like forward and side bends.

ANAL FISSURES

Often, constipation can be accompanied by anal fissures. Anal fissures are small tears or cracks in the lining of the anus. I can honestly say that these hurt worse than pushing a baby out of my vagina without pain management. Has the party started yet? Warm baths before a bowel movement with a tablespoon or two (15 to 30 ml) of coconut oil added to the warm water can help heal painful fissures, but hopefully you will be lucky enough to skip this less-than-desirable pregnancy side effect.

HEMORRHOIDS

Your pregnancy constipation can also lead to hemorrhoids. Hemorrhoids, aka piles, are swollen and inflamed veins located in the anus and rectum. They can bleed and itch, meaning they are literally a pain in the butt. If you skip them during pregnancy, you may still end up with them after pushing your baby out. Some can just be mildly uncomfortable, but I felt like I had sat on a shard of glass. Natural at-home remedies such as dabbing on apple cider vinegar or witch hazel helped ease my discomfort. Many of my doula clients talk to me about their hemorrhoids in a hushed and embarrassed tone. I let them know how incredibly common hemorrhoids are and that I am surprised when clients *don't* have any.

EXPERT TIP

on Hemorrhoids

by Robin Rose Bennett, *writer, green witch, herbalist, wisewoman, and founder of Wisewoman Healing Ways*

These are varicose veins in the anus. Drink plenty of water. Put your legs up the wall. Drink grape leaf and nettle infusions. Eat ½ cup (120 g) of cooked dark-colored berries such as blueberries, raspberries, or strawberries daily. Frozen ones work fine. Topically, use plantain (*Plantago major* or *lanceolata*) or witch hazel or yarrow oil or ointment, or a combination. Even drugstore witch hazel works, but it isn't as soothing.

on Hemorrhoid Relief

by Miracle Mattie, *my grandmother, herbalist, and massage therapist*

Pour apple cider vinegar onto a cotton ball and apply it to external piles a few times a day. For internal hemorrhoids, drink 1 teaspoon (15 ml) two to three times a day. You can also try rinsing the area with equal parts water and witch hazel using a perineal irrigation, or peri, bottle after each trip to the bathroom. This is great to have around post-delivery for helping heal after a vaginal delivery.

WEIGHT GAIN

Pregnancy weight gain varies depending on the person. During my first singleton pregnancy, I gained much more weight than I did when I was pregnant with my twins. Go figure! Each pregnancy is different, but that doesn't stop people from constantly telling us that we are either too big or too small. My advice is to ignore the people who make unsolicited comments about your pregnancy bump size. Your care provider is the only one whose opinion matters, so look there for guidance on healthy weight gain for your body during your pregnancy. Believe it or not, I miss my super curvy body and get serious bump envy when I spot a pregnant person. A doula client and dear friend of mine didn't gain much weight at all during her first pregnancy. Everyone, including her care provider, became very concerned. She had numerous ultrasounds during her pregnancy that all indicated that the baby was growing just fine. She gave birth to a perfectly healthy 7½-pound (3.4 kg) baby. Our bodies can carry babies very differently.

ADVICE FOR TRANSGENDER PREGNANT PARENTS-TO-BE

What happens when your pregnant body is being viewed as feminine by the public, but you identify as trans male, genderqueer, or non-feminine female? Being a transgender pregnant person can bring up mixed emotions while the pregnant body changes, the breasts enlarge, and the belly grows. Remind yourself that these changes are temporary, and they are part of the journey toward welcoming your new baby.

Trans men who become pregnant may have a difficult time finding compassionate care providers due to lack of awareness and support of pregnant men. Be easy on yourselves. You're doing amazing work. And FYI for those of you who don't know, an expecting person can be called *mom, dad, carrier,* or *gestational parent.*

I am damn proud of my warrior-mama tiger stripes! Believe it or not, I love them.

Reducing Anxiety During Pregnancy

FOR SOME PEOPLE, PREGNANCY CAN BE A BEAUTIFUL AND positive experience, while for others it can be filled with crippling anxiety. That anxiety can easily be fueled by the current trend in our country to instill fear and doubt about our body's natural ability to give birth— we are always hearing about all the things that can go wrong during pregnancy and childbirth. Instead of focusing on that, I want to share with you all the things that can go right. There is a fine balance between being fully informed and empowered, and reducing anxiety is key for having an empowered birth experience. In this chapter, I'll share a variety of techniques for calming your body and your mind.

MIND-BODY CONNECTION

The way we think, act, and feel can positively or negatively impact our biological functioning. In terms of childbirth, you give birth the way you live your life. My doula sisters and I at Carriage House Birth discuss this connection all the time. We write our own stories. We bear witness to this concept over and over again as birth doulas. Perhaps you should ask yourself, How do I act or respond in most situations? If you are

Unexpected Positivity

I was fortunate enough to support a doula client who ended up needing an unexpected but very necessary cesarean section while in labor. She was so excited to meet her baby that she surrendered her birth "plan" for an unmedicated vaginal delivery and embraced the journey that was unfolding. When I met her after the cesarean in the recovery room, she was glowing. She was radiating the most beautiful and bright, love-filled energy. Her baby (appropriately named Ocean) was on her chest skin-to-skin, and he was content. Her positivity and calm energy were definitely felt by this newborn soul. She taught me that you can have a positive birth experience even if it's not what you expected.

afraid and anxious most of the time, then your birth may be full of fear and, very likely, high blood pressure. If you are someone who prefers to embrace the "ignorance is bliss" philosophy, you will more than likely be shocked by the intensity of childbirth and perhaps suffer from post-traumatic stress disorder as a result. Whatever your normal mode, you can make conscious decisions before you give birth to work on some of your emotional baggage and less-than-desirable personality traits that can lead you to a challenging childbirth experience.

This certainly does *not* mean that if you have a difficult or traumatic birth that you somehow deserved that outcome or didn't put in the work. Perhaps there will be a silver lining in a traumatic childbirth experience that gives you an acute awareness and deeper understanding of life. My own childbirth trauma led me to become a birth doula.

SURRENDER

I love to compare labor contractions to ocean waves. If you stand in front of a huge wave and tense up your body and fight the wave, it's going to knock you flat on your ass. If you relax your body and surrender to the wave, you can actually ride over it. The less tension and anxiety you have, the easier the wave is to ride. If you feel stress, your baby feels stress. This can have a negative impact on your pregnancy and your childbirth. We cannot control exactly how our pregnancy or birth will unfold, but we can control how we feel about it. That's a lot of power. It's also a choice. We can choose to embrace chaos.

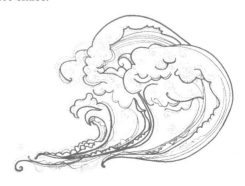

on Reducing Anxiety

by Robin Rose Bennett, *writer, green witch, herbalist, wisewoman, and founder of Wisewoman Healing Ways*

Lavender flower tea, 1 teaspoon per cup, brewed for 10 to 20 minutes, is delicious and soothing. Chamomile flower tea can be made similarly. Tincture of calming motherwort, 13 drops in a glass of tea or water, can also be used. Small amounts such as this are fine. Strong infusions could be too relaxing to the womb. A stronger, yet still safe, sedative herb is skullcap, and it can be used as a tincture, 7 to 10 drops in a glass of water or tea, or made as a simple tea, as above. Finally, one of my favorites is to boil 2 cups (75 g) of dried oatstraw herb in a half gallon (1.9 L) of water and then pour the herbs and water into a half gallon jar. Let steep for 8 hours. This soothing, mineral-rich brew can be drunk or poured (minus the herbs) into a bath. The only contraindication for this tea would be celiac disease.

PRENATAL YOGA

Prenatal yoga can be a great way to reduce anxiety and connect with your baby. It also prepares your body for labor by strengthening your uterus and pelvic floor. My favorite yoga pose during pregnancy and during labor was the cat/cow sequence. Kneel on all fours, belly drawn in. Inhale, drop your stomach, arch your back, and tilt your tailbone up toward the ceiling. Exhale and round your back as you tuck your chin to your chest. You will look like a pregnant cat stretching after a nap. Rock back and forth gently between these two poses. This will keep your spine loose and prevent stiffening. It can also be a wonderful tool during labor if you are experiencing back labor. I found that the focused breathing and the gentle stretching really helped ease my pregnancy anxiety.

on Prenatal Yoga

by Tara Stiles, *yoga instructor and founder of Strala Yoga*

Keeping or starting a regular, easygoing yoga practice during pregnancy is wonderful for easing anxiety, maintaining good energy levels, boosting mood and mental clarity, and cultivating a healthy, strong body. Try giving yourself twenty minutes each morning and a few moments before bed to allow your body to move through what feels good for that day. Allow your practice to be different each day depending on what your body is craving. Though your movements may vary, consistently doing yoga is key to feeling its awesome benefits, so keep it regular, even if only for a few moments each day. Your body and mind will thank you!

Back Labor

Back labor is intense lower back pain during the laboring process that comes with contractions or can remain constant throughout. This type of pain is usually caused by the pressure of your baby's head against your lower back.

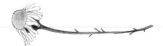

FIND A VILLAGE

Finding a community of expectant parents due around the same time as you can help you feel less alone in your childbearing journey. I was fortunate enough to find a welcoming group of folks, and sharing in the experience with them was a great stress reducer. Prenatal classes are available in many cities in the United States, and they are great places to start looking for some soon-to-be parents who are on the same timeline as you.

PRENATAL MASSAGE

Nothing takes the edge off of a stressful day quite like a good massage. Carrying around all that extra pregnancy weight can make your body feel sore and achy. These aches and pains can be soothed by the release of serotonin, your body's natural pain reliever, which is triggered by massage. Massage can also ease muscle tension and improve lymph and blood circulation. Break out that coconut oil for an anxiety-reducing self-massage or, even better, a rubdown from a partner or friend when you feel your tension level rising. There are also spas that cater to pregnant clientele with massage tables that have cut-out holes for growing bellies to rest in. After a good prenatal massage, I always had a good night's sleep, and few things are as anxiety-squashing as rest.

INTUITION

During pregnancy and childbirth, we are faced with many decisions. We decide where and how we would like to give birth. Then we make decisions once the baby is born regarding the infant's well-being and safety. Our intuition can help guide us in making good decisions. Intuition can also give insight with which to prepare ourselves emotionally. For instance, when I became pregnant a year and a half after I had my twin girls, I became obsessed with researching the chances of having two sets of twins. It's around one in three thousand. I had dreams that I was pregnant with twins again. My husband also *knew* intuitively that it was twins. My intuition told me it was two boys. Fast-forward to the first ultrasound, and sure enough it was twins *again*, and they were indeed twin boys! I think my intuition spared both me and my husband heart attacks.

One of my doula colleagues had a street psychic tell her that she was going to have twins one day. She held on to this prediction for many years. When she got pregnant for the second time, her intuition kicked in, and she began asking me a ton of twin pregnancy–related questions.

TAKING RITUAL BATHS

by Deborah "Mama Medicine" Hanekamp, seeress in the healing arts as an initiated Amazonian shaman, reiki master, and yogini

RITUAL BATH FOR PEACE

One season ends, a new one begins; one week ends, a new one begins; one life phase ends, a new one begins; one phase of human nature ends, a new one begins. During times of transition, we can get caught up in our heads, making plans and being just a bit too future-focused. This bath is designed to keep us centered in the presence of peace. Regardless of your spiritual background or beliefs, taking the time for self-care and focusing on peace will reduce anxiety and clear the mind.

Ingredients

1 cup (250 g) pink Himalayan sea salt
5 drops frankincense essential oil
5 drops lavender essential oil
Wildflowers (especially marigold and mugwort) to cover surface of tub
1 stick sacred palo (palo santo stick)
1 smoky quartz crystal
1 rose quartz crystal

Ritual

- Draw a warm bath, mix in the salt and essential oils, and sprinkle the flowers onto the water.
- Burn sacred palo around yourself and your bath.
- Step into the bath, and dunk your head under water.
- Place the smoky quartz on your solar plexus.
- Place the rose quartz on your heart.
- Inhale and see a green, golden light at the crown of your head.

- Exhale and see that green golden light encircling your being, offering you support, peace, and protection.
- Inhale and see the green golden light pull into your heart center, as you focus your mind on what you love most in this world.
- Exhale and see that green golden light surrounding you in the power of your own love.
- Repeat at least three more times. Feel the presence and peace you've created.
- When you are ready to end your bath, press your hands to your heart in gratitude.

RITUAL BATH TO BRIGHTEN UP

If you live in the northern hemisphere, the short days and long nights of winter may begin to weigh on your emotions. Although I encourage looking at this time of year as a time to celebrate sacred aloneness and looking within to find your inner light, sometimes you just need to brighten up! This bath is like lying on a quartz crystal beach, feeling the sun kiss your skin and listening to the soft sounds of Mama Ocean (well, almost). If you don't have all the ingredients, it's okay! Just use what you do have. Also, this can work as a wonderful foot bath.

Ingredients

1 cup (250 g) sea salt
5 drops white sage essential oil
5 drops lavender essential oil
Daisies and roses
1 candle (I like white, unscented candles)
1 cinnamon stick
1 amethyst
1 carnelian
1 Lemurian crystal

1 clear quartz crystal

Jasmine green tea

Ritual

- Draw a warm bath, add the salt and essential oils to the water, and sprinkle the flowers onto the water.

- Light your candle.

- From the flame, bless yourself with the smoke of the cinnamon stick.

- Place the amethyst, carnelian, and Lemurian crystal in the bathwater.

- Step into the bath, and dunk your head under water.

- Take three rounds of bhastrika, which is rapid-fire breathing done by forcefully inhaling and exhaling through the nose 36 times. Three rounds makes a total of 108 breaths.

- Place the clear quartz crystal and your own healing hands on your solar plexus, imagining a bright sun coming from within; this is your source.

- Soak in the shiny energy you've created and sing "This Little Light of Mine."

- Drink the tea as you soak in the bath.

- When you are ready to end your bath, press your hands to your heart in gratitude.

Her first ultrasound confirmed that her intuition and the street psychic were indeed right: She was pregnant with twins!

Always listen to your gut. It doesn't lie, and it won't lead you astray if you learn to trust it. It's knowing without knowing. Anxiety, however, can cloud your intuition and cause you to second-guess what you already know. Our busy day-to-day lives can also sometimes prevent us from slowing down enough to listen. Clearing away mental chatter can help you hear your inner voice. Take time for solitude, and allow yourself to dive deep and access your intuition. Mindfulness and meditation can be beginning steps toward tapping into your intuitive wisdom.

PREGNANCY MEDITATION

Meditation can relax the mind and the pregnant body and is an excellent tool for minimizing anxiety during pregnancy. Stay away from the things that trigger your anxiety, and instead invest your energy in developing a regular meditation practice. To get started, choose the same time every day and commit to a regular practice. I usually wake up early and start my day with a quick fifteen-minute meditation. Thirty minutes is optimal but can sometimes be hard to squeeze into a busy day. I set a reminder alert on my calendar so I won't forget.

Begin by sitting comfortably and closing your eyes. Breathe normally and focus on your breath. Check in with your body, starting from the soles of your feet and working your way all the up to the crown of your head. I like to repeat some of my favorite pregnancy mantras in my head.

Fact:
Around 24 weeks' gestation, your developing baby will hear noises from the outside world. Pretty neat, right?

I keep it very simple. Some examples are "I am strong," "I am brave," "I am love," and "I am growing and nurturing a new life." Please don't get caught up in worrying about doing it wrong. Committing the time to meditate is an act of self-love. You cannot mess this up. I promise. If you are struggling to develop a meditation practice, there are many wonderful options for guided meditations that you can download and listen to.

TALKING TO YOUR BABY

"Hello, little bean. I love you and can't wait to meet you." I was constantly chatting with my growing seedlings while pregnant. I'd even have full-on conversations with my tummy while out grocery shopping. I received a few crooked glances and stares! I wasn't fazed, though, because it was a way for me to bond with my unborn children way before actually meeting them in the flesh. It also really helped ease my pregnancy anxiety. I distinctly remember being super pregnant with my twin girls at a Willie Nelson concert, and my babies were both kicking me in the ribs (I like to think of it as dancing) to "On the Road Again." So don't hold back singing lullabies to your pregnant belly. Your baby hears you.

A doula client of mine liked to unwind at the end of each day by lying in bed singing and playing lullaby music for her baby bump. Singing can release endorphins and improve your mood, so why not? When her little one arrived earth-side, she swore the same lullaby music and singing worked like magic to soothe her baby to sleep.

EXERCISE WITH DAILY WALKS

Keeping active while pregnant is good for your body and can help with your sanity. Exercise releases the feel-good hormones endorphins, which help battle stress and anxiety. Walking for 30 minutes a day is the perfect cardiovascular exercise for pregnant folks. You don't need to purchase

BIRTHING TRADITIONS IN THE AFRICAN AMERICAN COMMUNITY

by Shafia M. Monroe, DEM, CDT, MPH, founder of the International Center for Traditional Childbearing (ICTC)

The art of birthing for African American women is embedded in the Southern traditions of the twentieth century's granny midwife, who provided love, massage, motherly advice, prayers, and fresh vegetables during the perinatal period. During this era, pregnant women experienced being rubbed with salves and oils, and being fussed over with talcum powder and floral water to ease their labor. New mothers were pampered during the postpartum period, which extended beyond forty days, receiving care from her mother, grandmother, partner, and the women of her extended family. The granny midwife would check in regularly to monitor the mother's recuperation. When the time was right, the midwife would lead the ritual of walking the mother and baby around the house to signify that they were strong enough to interact with the extended family and eventually the larger community.

Research shows that the disproportionately higher rate of African American infant and maternal mortality is a result of perinatal stress caused by systemic racism and micro-aggressions. Society can help reduce stress for pregnant African American women by helping to eliminate racism, validating their stories, empowering everyone with information, ensuring that birth practices are culturally competent, and linking the pregnant women and their partners to black birth workers and midwives. There is a groundswell of African American women reclaiming their birth experiences, with midwives, doula services, culturally specific breastfeeding support, out-of-hospital births, and advocacy for birth justice.

any special equipment or pay for a class. Grab your sneakers and a water bottle, and head out the door. You can walk all the way up through your ninth month of pregnancy and even get labor moving with a long stroll. This low-impact exercise choice is good for all shapes, sizes, and fitness levels. No excuses. (Well, except care provider–prescribed bedrest.) Get walking!

PAMPERING YOURSELF

You are amazing. You are growing a freaking human being! You deserve to be pampered, so learn how to pamper yourself while pregnant and teach your partner and friends how you want to be pampered.

Here are some simple suggestions that really worked for me: I took an Epsom salt bath at the end of every day throughout my entire pregnancy. I became addicted to my aromatherapy infuser and pampered my sense of smell any chance I got. Lavender is my favorite essential oil for creating calm.

Unfortunately, I didn't have too much time for spa days and leisurely lunches with friends, but I seriously recommend them. You can also do something as simple as making yourself a cup of tea and throwing on a favorite movie. Don't forget to remind yourself what an amazing feat it is to grow a baby.

Pampering

Here's the definition of pampering in case you don't normally take the time to practice this form of intense self-love:

"Pamper (*verb*): to give someone special treatment, making that person as comfortable as possible and giving them whatever they want." (*Cambridge Dictionary*)

ALL-INCLUSIVE PREGNANCY AND CHILDBIRTH

Families comes in all different shapes, sizes, colors, and genders. When it comes to giving birth to and caring for a newborn, there is a large range of family dynamics, conception journeys, gender issues, and parenting philosophies to explore. I encourage the LGBTQIA families that I work with to consider seeking out a childbirth education class geared specifically toward queer families. The value of being heard and accepted in a safe space with other families navigating their childbearing journey is tremendous.

The vast disparities in health statistics along race lines in the United States are very alarming. According to the Centers for Disease Control and Prevention, black women are four times more likely to die during pregnancy or childbirth than white women. This disparity stretches across all levels of income, age, and education. Research indicates that stress is a huge factor in these negative outcomes, and stress is often triggered by racial discrimination. The physiological response to chronic stress helps explain the racial disparities in birth outcomes. Compassionate, evidence-based care needs to become readily available for every global citizen to be able to improve these outcomes.

The ugly reality is that many people are being treated differently by their care providers and medical establishments based on the color of their skin, their socioeconomic status, and their gender identity. We deserve better. We must start to demand better. People need to really work on changing the current climate of ignoring and denying the racism, homophobia, and patriarchy that poison the maternal health care system for our pregnant global citizens. This is a human rights issue. If we can change the way we treat people when they give birth, we can change the world for the better. I believe that deeply in my soul.

Naming Your Baby

I CHOSE THE NAMES MIA, BIRDIE AND HAZEL (TWINS), LUKE and Rocco (twins), and Olympia for my children. Naming my babies was an enjoyable process. I loved researching and trying on all the different names. I would have ten more babies if my husband would let me, just to use up my favorite baby names. Just kidding. Well, sort of.

How do you pick a baby name that you won't end up regretting? The name you choose will only last a lifetime—no pressure! It can be overwhelming to choose the perfect name. Many people name their children after family members. Honoring a family tradition may be something that is extremely important to you. It was important to me. Most of my children have a middle name that honors a relative, and I was honored when my nephew was given my first name as his middle name. Thank goodness he's a real firecracker and living up to his namesake. I had a client who named her baby after her mother, but she didn't announce it until the family was gathered in the hospital room after the birth. There was not a dry eye in the room!

Here are a few suggestions for beginning the process if you haven't already selected a name.

Nowadays there are a slew of baby naming websites that you can get lost in. The names are usually grouped under categories such as popular names, celebrity baby names, or vintage names. You can also find baby name books online or at your local bookstore. I loved curling up in bed with a cup of tea, some raw chocolate, and a highlighter for picking top baby name contenders. I tend to really gravitate toward vintage-sounding names, and my research led me to the Social Security Administration website to view the most popular names according to year. It's a great resource for inspiration. Somewhere between 1920 and 1930, I found my twin daughters' names, Birdie and Hazel. Other folks go off the beaten path altogether to find a name that feels right. I had clients choose Flash as the name for their son, and although I've heard a ton of unique baby names, that one really stands out.

The way I named my last daughter was a completely different process altogether. One of my close friends had named her daughter by simply asking her. What? Sounds easy, right? She explained that she had a baby naming ceremony in which she asked the baby, while she was still in the womb, what her name was. I was fascinated and jumped at the chance when she offered to hold a baby naming ceremony for me and my growing baby. I was skeptical that a name would come up because my husband and I had already decided pretty definitively on the name Pearl. During the ceremony, I entered into a meditative state and asked my baby what her name was. Nothing happened for a few minutes, and then, loud and clear, the name *Olympia* came through. I had never even considered the name before and wasn't even sure that I liked it. I set my ego aside and truly believed that my daughter had picked her name. Convincing my husband was challenging, but he eventually came around. So Olympia it is. Pretty magical, right?

The one thing that may shock you during this naming process is that people are very quick to give you their negative responses to your name choices. Of course, if you are asking for their honest response, that's one thing, but most of the time you're just answering the question that pregnant women get asked again and again while pregnant: "What are you naming the baby?" With my first baby, I got nothing but positive responses from friends and family. I can't help but wonder if this was only because of the popularity of the name Mia. During my second pregnancy, I was left with the overwhelming task of naming not just one but two baby girls. Everyone had something to say about my choices, and most were negative. What people had to say didn't sway my opinion, but it did really irritate me when friends and family would flat-out say, "I don't like that." I wanted to say, "Wow, really? Because that's what I'm naming them, so deal with it."

You may hear a list of reasons why the name sounds like an old lady name or why your child will be made fun of in school. The thing about uncommon or different names is that today, especially in Brooklyn, uncommon is common. I know a few little girls with the name Birdie. In that same neighborhood, my daughter went to school with two kids named Bowie and played with a handful of children named Blue and

Meditate to Find a Name

- Find a quiet and peaceful place to sit comfortably for approximately 15 to 20 minutes.
- If inside, light some candles and dim the lights.
- Focus on your breath. Place one hand on your heart and the other hand on your belly. Bring awareness to each part of your body starting at your toes. Move up the entire body and release any tension that you may be holding.
- Image yourself in nature. Where do you feel the most peaceful and connected to the earth? I imagined myself walking into the middle of a lush forest surrounded by massive redwood trees.
- Now ask your baby what their name is. You may hear a name loud and clear, or you may only get a letter. Listen to your baby.

Wolf. I advise you to ignore what anyone says in regard to naming your babies. It will only get you angry and make you question what you know in your heart is the right choice. When you're telling people the name you've chosen, you can even preface it by letting them know you aren't asking for their opinion. Now, here are some names that I didn't end up using, so have at them!

Girls: Adelaide, Beatrice, Bunny, Cinnamon, Clementine, Coraline (Cora), Cordelia, Eloise, Fern, Flora, Freyja, Ginger, Ida, Imogen, Ivy, Josephine (Joey), Magnolia (Maggie), Maisie, Marcela, Marigold (Goldie), Marilyn, Nova, Olive, Pearl, Penelope (Penny), Pepper, Poppy, Skye, Sparrow, Tallulah, Tilly, Tulip, Valentine, Violet, Vita, Vivienne, Winifred (Winnie), Winona, and Wren.

Boys: Alden, Bear, Benny, Bruno, Butch, Caleb, Carmine, Caspar, Chet, Clem, Cosmo, Floyd, Freedom (Free), Geno, Hart, Ike, James, Lemuel, Leo, Leroy, Louis (Louie), Mateo, Monty, Moss, Nash, Otis, Otto, Phoenix, Poe, Rene, River, Rufus, Sergio, Skye, Sonny, Stone, Tanner, Theo, True, Valentine, Vinny, Vito, and Walter.

Assembling Your Support Team

SUPPORT TEAM? IS CHILDBIRTH A GROUP SPORT? THERE
are many expectant parents who may wonder why they would need or
even want a support team. Don't you just go to the hospital and pop out
a baby? How hard could it be? I wish it were this easy. Honestly, with my
first baby, I was in complete and total denial that the act of giving birth
would be that big a deal. Haven't we been giving birth since the beginning of time? The thing is, I was wrong. Very, very, very, very wrong.

Giving birth for the first time shook me to the core. It blasted me
open both literally and figuratively. It was the biggest deal I was ever put
up against. The experience showed me that having a support team during
your childbearing journey is of utmost importance. Here's why: It truly
takes a village. A 2012 Cochrane Review found that continuous support during pregnancy and childbirth results in better outcomes. (The
Cochrane Database of Systematic Reviews is the leading resource for
systematic reviews in health care. Cochrane evidence will enhance your
health care knowledge and will aid in important decision making during
your pregnancy.)

Although you don't need to do this alone if you don't want to, I'm
not suggesting that you should invite a large group of people onto your
support team—unless that's what makes you feel more supported. Here
are a few people who may be essential to creating your birth team: your
partner (if applicable), a family member, a best friend, your care provider, and perhaps a birth doula.

Your support team should help you before, during, and after the
birth of your baby or babies. You should all meet a few times prenatally to
discuss your birthing preferences. It helps to have everyone on the same
page. Your support team will remain by your side during the laboring
process, whether it's two hours or three days long. We've got you. Once
your wee one comes earth-side, it's a good idea to call on this support
team for those first postpartum weeks. Don't hesitate to tell your village
if you need support. It's one thing I wish I had done sooner in my own
childbearing journey.

> **dou·la**
>
> *noun* A person who is trained to assist another person during childbirth and who may provide support to the family after the baby is born.

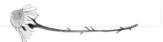

WHAT IS A DOULA?

I get asked this question frequently when I tell people what my job title is. Often people confuse doulas with midwives. Doulas don't catch babies or offer medical advice. We are strictly concerned with the waist up. Nowadays, though, I get asked this question less because so many celebrities are utilizing the services of a doula. To answer the question above, I usually respond with, "I'm a childbirth coach." This sums it up so almost anyone can understand it. Obviously, I know that what we offer is much, much more than just a labor coach, but it's my short answer for people who probably don't want to hear me ramble on about the amazing role I have during childbirth.

The word *doula* comes from the ancient Greek meaning "a woman who serves" and is now used to refer to a trained and experienced professional (regardless of gender) who provides continuous physical, emotional, and informational support to the person giving birth before, during, and just after birth; or who provides emotional and practical support during the postpartum period.

HOLDING SPACE

Your ideal support person (maybe it's a partner or a birth doula) will hold space for you. What does it mean to hold space for another person? It means to walk alongside someone and give unwavering, nonjudgmental support. Your space holders shouldn't be trying to fix you or make suggestions for you based on themselves or their egos. They should allow you to step into your own power if you so choose. Your support people create a safe space for you to process lots of really big and intense emotions while still being held. They can help you organize what may feel like chaos during your birth. This is one of the biggest assets to having a support team.

THE BENEFIT OF HAVING A BIRTH DOULA

Some people think that a doula is only for the new-agey types and not for modern-day folk. This couldn't be further from the truth. Doulas are for *everyone*. (Disclaimer: I do own Birkenstocks and love crystals.) Studies have shown that when doulas attend birth, labors are shorter with fewer complications, babies are healthier, and they breastfeed more easily. Not bad, huh?

I attend births in the hospital, at birthing centers, and in people's homes. My goal is for a pregnant person and their partner (if applicable) to have an informed birth. Knowledge is power. I have no other agenda. No doula should judge you or make you feel bad for the choices you make during your birth. We are there to be your advocate. Cost should not be a deterrent, either. Many doulas-in-training offer free or dis-counted services. I always make a point to weave in pro bono clients with my paying clients.

Another very popular misconception is that doulas are only for people who want an unmedicated vaginal birth. I work with clients who plan on getting an epidural but would like some tips and techniques for managing labor at home before heading to the hospital. I also have assisted clients through planned cesarean births. If you are hoping for an unmedicated birth, a doula will definitely increase your chances of having one, but your doula will be there for you no matter what birthing

on Doula Support

by Village Obstetrics, *obstetrician-gynecologist practice in New York City*

Doula support is an essential tool for a satisfying birth experience, especially for VBAC, unmedicated birth, and first birth.

plan you choose. Every birth is different, and having a knowledgeable advocate throughout the process is a huge asset.

A birthing partner may worry that a doula will take over during the birth. This should never be the case. We are often the doula for partners as well, making sure they are fed, caffeinated, and rested so they can be the best possible birth partner for the laboring person. We can also take some pressure off of the partner as the primary birth partner and help normalize the process. This can reduce anxiety for everyone involved. I describe a doula during the birthing process as a family member without all the family drama, hang-ups, and judgment. We help produce from the sidelines. I vividly recall one birth in which my clients labored beautifully as a team and wanted me to hang out in another room. Occasionally they would call out to me that they needed water or that they wanted me to time the labor contractions from my station. Later they told me that I was extremely helpful in normalizing the process for them and that it really allowed for them to labor intimately with one another without fear and anxiety.

BLIND DATING WITH DOULAS: FIVE TIPS ON FINDING *THE ONE!*

Considering hiring a birth doula? Great! Now how do you actually go about choosing someone to support you on the most intimate, vulnerable, and life-changing journey of your entire life? No small task. I'm hoping that I can make this somewhat nerve-racking matchmaking easier for you (and perhaps your partner). At this point, you have reached out to a few potential doulas and set up your free consultations. Okay . . .

1   Does the doula make you feel at ease when discussing your upcoming birth? Your doula should normalize the birthing process and help you remain calm and focused on birthing your baby. Certain energies/personalities do not mesh well, while others click right away.

2   Ask your potential doula, "Why did you chose to become a birth doula?" It's a wonderful icebreaker and may help you understand their personality and approach to childbirth. My passion for this work always seems to bubble over when people ask me this question.

3   Know what you are looking for in a birth doula. What type of requirements do you feel are important to support you best through your birth? Some clients want experience in body work, aromatherapy, or yoga. Some clients are looking for doulas who are mothers or who specialize in twin pregnancies and/or vaginal births after cesarean.

4   Know your budget. The cost of doula services range from free to $3,000 and up. Many of these fees are based on experience level and additional training. Every expecting person deserves affordable labor support. Many doulas offer payment plans and sliding-scale fees. I personally love the ancient art of bartering. I recently attended a birth in exchange for mixed martial arts classes for my kids. Score!

5   Trust your gut. Finding the right doula is about personality as much as it is about training and common understanding. Does your potential doula give you excited butterflies? If so, that's the one.

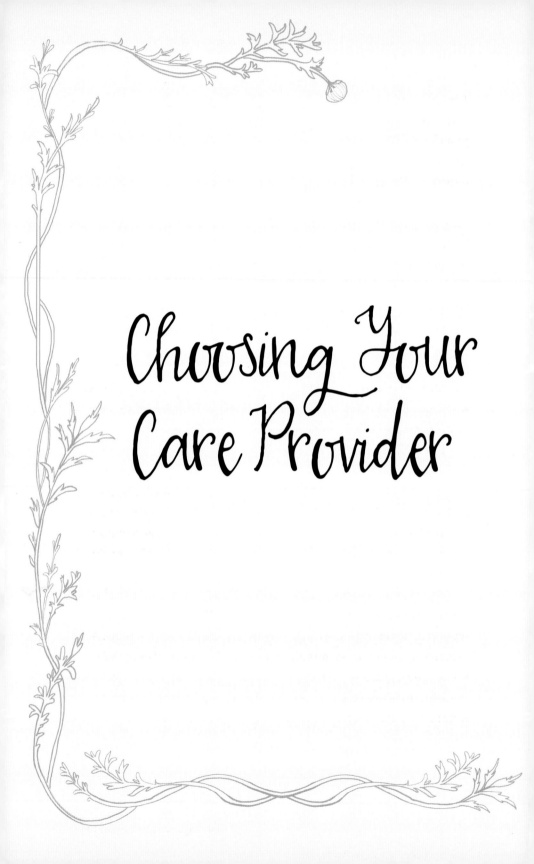

Choosing Your Care Provider

THE MOST IMPORTANT DECISION THAT YOU WILL MAKE IN your childbearing journey is who your care provider will be. Your care provider will be guiding you in making medical decisions for yourself and your baby. Having confidence in your birthing body and in your care provider will enable you to have a safe and healthy childbirth.

Hire a care provider for skill and experience but also, please, like your care provider. It will be much easier to ask questions and receive feedback from a care provider you like and trust. Yes, you can have the best of both worlds. You deserve both.

Here are some examples of cases in which you should find a new care provider as soon as possible: "My OB is very busy and rarely answers any of my questions," and "I don't really like my care provider, but I guess that's not really important." *Wrong*! It's very important. People plan for major life events (like weddings) for months or even years and pay attention to every single detail. You wouldn't keep a wedding planner who didn't have time to answer your questions, so why should the care provider for the birth of your child be treated any differently?

I strongly recommend interviewing a few different care providers to find an appropriate match based on your birthing preferences. You are the consumer. Please don't forget that. You can have the most amazing partner and/or birth doula and still have a negative birth experience due to a misaligned care provider. Your care provider will ultimately be making decisions for you and your baby if anything goes wrong. Your safety and your baby's safety should be in trusted hands.

A person aiming to have an unmedicated childbirth may not be best matched with a high-risk obstetrician. Interviewing a midwife who has supported numerous unmedicated deliveries would be a better route. A preexisting condition (such as high blood pressure, heart disease, diabetes, or epilepsy) can require an obstetrician or a maternal fetal medicine specialist to deliver your baby. But even with a high-risk pregnancy, you will still have choices, so please find a doctor you connect with.

MIDWIVES AND OBSTETRICIANS

Now it's time to choose your care provider. Midwife or obstetrician? What's the difference? Obstetrician gynecologists, or OB/GYNs, are medical doctors who specialize in the management of pregnancy, labor, and birth. They are trained to detect and manage obstetrical and gynecological problems. They are also trained to perform cesarean sections. In many urban areas, they work in large practices and cannot offer a continuous model of care, meaning you roll the dice; you don't know which doctor in the practice will be catching your baby. This can be stressful for some clients. If financially possible, I encourage my clients to explore a solo practitioner or an OB/GYN practice that only has two doctors. The small obstetrics practices offer a personalized care model that allows for a trusting relationship to form. It may really put you at ease to know the doctor who will be there for you on your delivery day.

A midwife is a trained medical professional who assists in the pregnancy, labor, and delivery of healthy expectant people. The midwifery approach is often very different from contemporary obstetrical care. Midwives offer a personalized and holistic approach to childbirth. Your emotional and physical well-being are important to your midwife. Midwives believe that birth is a natural process and intervene only if medically necessary.

Midwives

According to an April 2016 Cochrane Review, women who received midwife-led continuity models of care were less likely to experience intervention and more likely to be satisfied with their care with at least comparable adverse outcomes for women or their infants than women who received other models of care. In other words, women who receive hands-on care from midwives have better births. Having a care provider who is supporting you throughout your childbirth journey is important to women.

CHOOSING YOUR BIRTHING PLACE

To determine where you want to deliver your baby, you should first assess your birthing needs. Are you having a high-risk pregnancy? Do you require being in a hospital to deliver your baby? If you are not deemed high risk and you are having a healthy pregnancy, you will have more options for where you can potentially deliver, such as at a birthing center or in your house.

I work as a birth doula in hospitals, birthing centers, and clients' homes, and I have also been fortunate enough to deliver my own children in all these settings. Each experience was different, and each has many pros and cons. One of the most important factors in deciding on a place to birth your baby is your overall feeling of safety. For my first birth, I felt the safest at an in-hospital birthing center. My most recent birth was in my home, and it felt like it was the safest choice for me and my baby.

Do your research. Find out what your birthing options are for where you live. Different hospitals also have different policies surrounding childbirth. For instance, you may not be able to have a water birth in most hospital settings. Take some tours, talk to friends, and perhaps pick the brain of a doula in your local community to find the appropriate birthing location for you and your baby.

EVIDENCE-BASED CARE

Evidence-based care utilizes current scientific evidence and focuses on the individual needs of the clients to make informed decisions regarding their care. Unfortunately, most care providers and hospitals in the United States do *not* practice evidence-based care. The core of this problem may lie in the education and training practices of physicians and nurses. The focus is primarily on what can go wrong during childbirth. This type of training is very important, but it doesn't focus enough on how to facilitate a normal, uncomplicated vaginal delivery.

I can only speak from my personal experience as a birth doula, but I have encountered numerous obstetricians and labor and delivery nurses who rarely witness and are surprised by an uninterrupted physiological birth. Many are baffled when a client declines an epidural and wants to be out of the hospital bed. My definition of *uninterrupted birth* is not having continuous fetal monitoring, having no IV, eating during labor at will, and moving freely during the process. These types of births are typically not included in their education process. This seems to be a bigger systematic problem.

I believe that the safety of the birthing person and the baby is always of utmost importance. I also believe that the emotional well-being of the birthing person and the baby is *also* very important and often neglected. This holistic model of care has been proven to reduce instances of postpartum depression. Why is this such a hard concept to grasp? Perhaps many institutions are just set in their ways and their routines.

In 2015, the American Society of Anesthesiologists came out with a study saying that most people in labor would benefit from a light meal. (My assumption is that this would not include people who have scheduled a surgical birth.) There have been many improvements made to the anesthesia that is being used for pain management during childbirth, which reduces the risk for eating while in labor. Regardless of these recent studies, though, many hospitals still only allow ice chips during labor. It's proof that evidence-based care is not always practiced.

Here are a few questions that you can ask your potential care providers to see if they practice evidence-based care and if they are an appropriate fit for you. (See pages 198 and 199 for a version of this list you can copy and write on.)

○ Do you practice evidence-based care?
○ What are your philosophies surrounding pregnancy, labor, and childbirth?
○ What is your cesarean rate? (A lower rate is typically better, as most people are hoping to avoid a surgical delivery. If you are planning a

cesarean, there's no need to be concerned; the cesarean rate is at an all-time high, so most practices are very experienced.)

- ○ Do you routinely induce clients at a certain number of weeks pregnant?
- ○ Do you routinely cut episiotomies? (An episiotomy is a surgical cut in the perineum, the area between the vagina and the anus, made to enlarge the vaginal opening for delivery. This used to be a routine procedure many years ago and is now only used in certain cases.)
- ○ Do you routinely rupture the bag of waters?
- ○ What other standard routine practices should I expect?
- ○ Who will be my care provider if you are not on call for my delivery?
- ○ How do you feel about doulas?
- ○ Do you have a time limit on the length of labor?
- ○ Can I room in with my baby (meaning have your baby stay in your room as opposed to the nursery)?
- ○ Is the hospital baby/family friendly?

THE THREE P'S

Learning the three P's, *policies*, *procedures*, and *politics*, will help you navigate your childbearing journey with knowledge and assertiveness.

In choosing where to give birth, you must consider the policies that are in place. Hospitals and birthing centers are bound by their policy protocols, which means that you will be, too. In New York City, for example, many of my clients are surprised to discover that the partner is unable to stay after the baby is born unless a private room is purchased. Typically, private rooms are very expensive and are often booked up. Doing research beforehand will help prevent surprises like this at your place of birth.

Procedures during pregnancy and childbirth include routine and non-routine prenatal testing, interventions during labor, and newborn

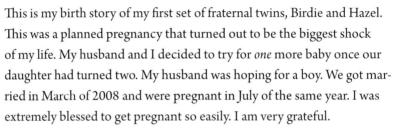

MY SECOND BIRTH

Birdie Elaine and Hazel Marilyn
March 19, 2009
Twin Hospital Birth

This is my birth story of my first set of fraternal twins, Birdie and Hazel. This was a planned pregnancy that turned out to be the biggest shock of my life. My husband and I decided to try for *one* more baby once our daughter had turned two. My husband was hoping for a boy. We got married in March of 2008 and were pregnant in July of the same year. I was extremely blessed to get pregnant so easily. I am very grateful.

I really wanted to have a home birth this time around. I decided to go to my regular OB to get an initial scan of the baby before meeting with a midwife. At 10 weeks, I went in and got an ultrasound.

"There's only one, right?" I said, totally kidding.

"Oh my gosh, there's two!" my OB said.

Twins? Holy crap! Shock turned into excitement. I called my husband Dan, and he thought I was pulling his chain.

I then became unsure about our birth plan. We really didn't have one anymore. We found a home birth midwife who said she would still deliver me at home, but I had some apprehension. I really needed to examine all my options and all the risks associated with twins. *Wow*! Reluctantly, I gave up on the home birth plan and decided to deliver in a hospital as naturally and drug free as possible. I went on the hunt for a badass doula who could be a sounding board for me and my husband in the operating room. The standard procedure in New York City is to deliver twins in the operating room. I was not too fond of that part, but I understood that it was for safety reasons. I spoke with my OB, and she told us that the doula could be in the laboring room but not the operating room. She wasn't too keen on the idea of a doula. I decided reluctantly that Dan would be my primary support person.

The OB also strongly suggested an epidural if I was hoping for a vaginal birth. At thirty-five weeks, I went to my OB and she said that all looked good. Both babies were in the vertex position. She said it might be a few days or weeks; it's hard to tell with twins. I was in constant pain from the weight of the babies. I had put on 40 to 50 pounds (18 to 22 kg) at this point. Little did I know that I would go into labor a day later.

I woke up with some cramps. I first thought it might have been the burger that I had for dinner. My husband was convinced that this was not labor. It was around 7 a.m., and the contractions became consistent almost immediately. They were three minutes apart right from the get-go. I knew at that point that we needed to head to the hospital. I was nervous that it would be as quick as my previous birth with Mia.

The experience in the hospital was very different from my previous experience in a birthing center within a hospital. I was checked and admitted. I think I was around 6 to 7 cm dilated. I got the epidural pretty quickly because they insisted on constant fetal monitoring. I couldn't move from the bed. I also kept knocking off the monitors while I was contracting. My labor slowed down once I got the epidural. I have a feeling that if I hadn't gotten it, I would have delivered very quickly. I was in labor about eight hours total, so it was still pretty quick. The OB who was on call to deliver my girls offered a cesarean section because of their size difference. I declined, saying I would only get one in an emergency.

Once I was fully dilated, they wheeled me into the operating room. I pushed for fifteen minutes and at 3:06 p.m. Birdie came out easily. The OB applied fundal pressure and I pushed out Hazel at 3:12 p.m. She came out sunny-side up. I was able to nurse them right away, and they had no health issues from being born at thirty-five weeks and three days. Hazel weighed 6 pounds, 7 ounces (2.9 kg) and Birdie was my peanut at 5 pounds, 8 ounces (2.5 kg). I was in a daze for the first few days. Holy crap, I just had twins! I love my girls and was so grateful that they were born vaginally and healthy. I must admit that I hated giving birth in a hospital. My anxiety was high, and it contributed to intensifying my labor pains. This experience is what inspired me to become a doula. I knew that birthing twins could be done naturally at home (though it shouldn't always be). I didn't know that I would have a chance to give it go again a few short years later with my second set of twins.

care procedures. You can research the most up-to-date prenatal testing that is offered during your pregnancy. Many of these tests are optional and others are strongly recommended by your care provider. Please weigh the pros and cons of these tests and decide what's best for you and your baby. When it comes to intervention procedures, again, knowledge is important. Take a childbirth education class to understand the reasons behind using interventions during labor. Some interventions are necessary for your and your baby's safety, and other interventions are completely optional. You can always ask, "Am I okay," "Is my baby okay," and "Do we have time to think about it?" Many states and cities have mandatory newborn procedures. For example, in most hospitals it is mandatory to give a newborn the vitamin K injection. It's given because newborns are born with a low level of vitamin K, which is responsible for preventing a hemorrhage. Antibiotic eye ointment is also mandatory in many places to prevent the transmission of sexually transmitted diseases from a birthing person to the baby. What are the required newborn procedures where you live? What can you opt out of? What are the pros and cons? Knowledge will give you the power to make the right choices for your new baby.

The politics of birth refer to the way our society and culture view and feel about birth. We have a culture of judging everyone's choices. You're either too small or too fat. You probably shouldn't be eating or drinking that. You're insane to want an epidural-free birth! Shall I keep going? The media also teach us to fear birth. That fear then benefits medical and pharmaceutical companies because we seek stuff we don't need. More fear means more prenatal testing, extra ultrasounds, and more doctor visits that may not be medically necessary.

Navigating through the three P's of giving birth today will help you create individualized birthing preferences that are right for you, whether you are at home, a birth center, a hospital, or wherever you find the most comfort.

Choosing a Birthing Method/ Childbirth Education Class

I STRONGLY ENCOURAGE ALL EXPECTANT FOLKS AND their partners to take a childbirth education class. Knowing your options in childbirth will enable you to have choices. If you don't know your choices, then you don't have any! As a birth doula, I'm reluctant to work with clients who are not willing to educate themselves on the process. I'm just the doula; I can't birth the baby for them. You need to know the basics of what to expect, or you may find yourself bewildered during what is already a very intense experience. Now that I have convinced you that it is absolutely essential to take a childbirth education class, which class should you take?

Before you pick a class, my first recommendation is to take a childbirth class in person. It is really nice to be around other people who are experiencing the childbirth journey at the same time you are. You are not obligated to make lifelong buddies, so there's no pressure, either. My husband was worried he'd have to roll around on the floor and massage complete strangers. This did not happen. It was a nice way to take a pause from our busy lives and focus on the fact that we were having a baby. It helps to lift that heavy fog of denial. Any time after thirty-two weeks is a good time to take a class. You don't want to take it too early and forget all those juicy nuggets of wisdom.

There are a bunch of different childbirth education class options. You can find a local one by searching online or asking a friend. Your care provider will be able to direct you to classes, but know that hospital birthing classes may promote their own policies and slant toward teaching you how to be a good patient.

So how do you find a class that is right for you? Start by asking yourself what type of birthing experience you would like. What tools are you planning to use to manage the intensity of labor? Are you having a planned surgical birth? Do you have a hands-on partner? Do you want to go to a hospital or have a home birth? This will help you pick a class.

THE BRADLEY METHOD OF NATURAL CHILDBIRTH

The Bradley Method views birth as a natural process and teaches unmedi-cated childbirth. The partner is the coach and is heavily relied on for labor support. It emphasizes healthy eating, breathing, exercises, relaxation, and education. A little fun fact: my mother was a Bradley childbirth instructor when I was growing up, and she would teach expectant couples in our living room. I knew what a uterus was at the ripe age of two.

HYPNOBIRTHING

The hypnobirthing philosophy is that nature has intended for us to give birth relatively easily, and it is fear that causes pain. The idea is to replace fear with relaxation. Hypnobirthing uses visualization, affirmations, and self-hypnosis soundtracks. Hypnobirthing relaxation techniques also have tremendous value if an unexpected (or planned) cesarean birth becomes necessary.

THE LAMAZE METHOD

This is a prepared childbirth technique founded by French obstetrician Fernand Lamaze in the 1940s. Today, Lamaze is one of the leading childbirth education classes. It teaches labor coping techniques, comfort measures, relaxation, movement, and massage. *Hee hee hoo. Hee hee hoo.* That signature patterned breathing technique is no longer taught in most modern Lamaze classes. Too bad, right?! Breath work can be a wonderful coping tool for pregnant and laboring people. Breathing can become an automatic response to pain during labor. There are many yoga practi-tioners and breath workers who host workshops that use breath work as an active meditation technique to help reduce anxiety. There are also online resources if you are interested in learning pattered breathing.

Natural vs. Unmedicated

The term *natural childbirth* is antiquated. Let's use the term *unmedicated birth*. I hate that if you use an epidural or have a surgical delivery, it is considered unnatural or abnormal. Well, not in this book!

CARRIAGE HOUSE BIRTH CHILDBIRTH EDUCATION

Carriage House Birth offers a holistic approach to the childbearing journey. It embraces elements from many various birthing methods to create an extremely well-rounded curriculum. Normalizing childbirth for the expectant families is the goal of Carriage House Birth. The only downside is that you can't benefit from their amazing classes in person unless you live in New York City. But fear not, you can download a Carriage House Birth childbirth education class and watch and learn from the comfort of your own home.

SPECIALIZED CLASSES

There are also plenty of specialized childbirth classes, such as LGBTQIA Childbirth Education, Childbirth Education for Home Births, Birthing from Within ("birth-in-awareness"), Twin Prep (I teach a twin prep class called Twin Magic), VBAC Prep, Yoga for Labor, and many more options.

Now go sign up for a childbirth education class, and get psyched! You will be able to make informed decisions for you and your baby during your birthing journey. You are one step closer to a radical birth experience!

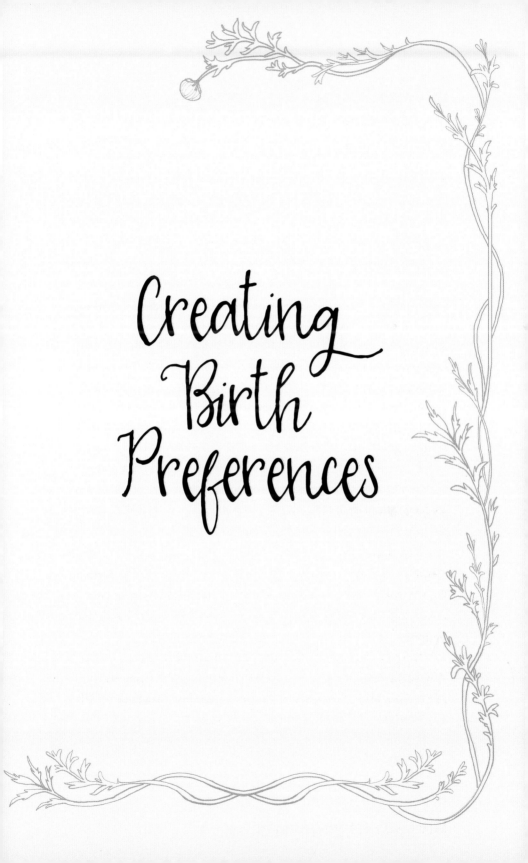

Creating Birth Preferences

YOU MAY NOTICE THAT I AM NOT CALLING THIS SECTION *Birth Plan*. I am using the word *preferences* instead. As much as we may want our birth to go a certain way, we cannot fully plan on how the experience will unfold. That said, we can plan as much as possible by discussing all the what-ifs. It is a good idea to start by highlighting your birth priorities. Keep it short and simple. It is a good exercise for you and your support team to create and discuss your preferences so you are all on the same page.

Unfortunately, many birthing families who utilize and hand out a birth plan in a medical setting will get sideways glances from the hospital staff. They may only glance at your plan or preferences without much thought. They may even whisper and comment about the laboring person "signing up for a C-section" when toting a birth plan. The staff is making the assumption that the family is inflexible and only wants to be defensive. Don't let this deter you. Know how you feel about all the possibilities. The people who refuse to consider all the what-ifs are usually the ones that have very unexpected and traumatic birth outcomes. If your biggest fear is a surgical delivery, my advice would be to research family-centered cesarean births (see below) and educate yourself on your options if this mode of delivery becomes necessary. Dive in where you are uncomfortable. It's the only way to move past it and have a positive birth experience. This is your birth, and you are the consumer. You

Family-Centered Cesarean

A family-centered cesarean is a cesarean birth during which the hospital staff helps the birthing family mimic what happens during a natural childbirth. This is facilitated by initiating a few requests from the family that may include immediate skin-to-skin contact, keeping a calm atmosphere, delayed cord clamping, and immediate breastfeeding if the birthing parent desires.

on Childbirth

by Elizabeth Bachner, *midwife and owner of GraceFull Birth*

There is a myth out there that birth is a line. A physical line that can be controlled and has set markers and time limits that always mean the same thing. The challenge with this perception is that it caters to the world where black-and-white thinking is thought to be ideal; the world where there are perpetual problems that need to be fixed and perfectionism is a goal. Childbirth, when left to communicate its unique journey, is not a straight line that goes from point A to point B; rather, it is a bunch of wheels, like those of a clock, each turning in unison, connected to the other, with its own unique layers of physical, mental, emotional, and spiritual ways in which we live our individualized lives.

deserve a positive birth whether your little one enters the world through the door or the window.

I had one determined client write up the most ironclad birth preferences document I have ever seen. She even got the hospital administration to sign off on some of her requests. She really worked hard to ensure that her wishes were heard and respected. Her birth unfolded beautifully, and the care provider and hospital staff were very respectful of her requests. This is an instance in which the birthing preference document was completely essential to having the client's wishes be heard.

THINGS TO INCLUDE IN YOUR BIRTH PREFERENCES

The first thing to do when you begin putting together your preferences is to explore all the policies and procedures that are standard at your place of delivery. Discuss these policies with your care provider so you can be fully informed and prepared. I've had clients switch from the hospital where they were planning on giving birth to a completely different hospital that better accommodated their birthing wishes. If you want an uninterrupted water birth, for example, a labor and delivery floor in the hospital more than likely won't accommodate your wishes. Know what's on the menu where you are delivering.

Now, who's on the guest list? Do you have a partner, a birth doula, a friend, and/or a family member who is part of your birth support team? Make sure you know your care provider's policy on how many people can assist you during your birth. A red flag for you may be that your care provider doesn't allow you to have a doula present. It's never too late to switch practices. Well it could be, but it's never too late to try.

Here's the topic that everyone loves to discuss: to epidural or not to epidural. What are your goals for managing the intensity of your labor? It's best to think this through ahead of time, because you know what really bugs me? I hate (strong word, I know) when care providers and/or nurses scare clients into getting an epidural. They taunt them by saying, "Oh, you think it's bad now, well it's going to get much worse" or "No one gives you a medal to do it without an epidural." The majority of the doula clients I work with are grown-ups. They also know that epidurals are on the menu at the hospital. They're not walking into an Italian restaurant and wondering if they serve pasta. You can ask for an epidural if you want one. You can also do it without an epidural. Whatever you decide for managing the intensity of your labor, make sure you share your preferences with your support team and your care provider.

Many of my doula clients like having a safe word, such as *watermelon*, *spaceship*, or *motorcycle*, for requesting an epidural. If the laboring person says the word, I know we should get that anesthesiologist as quickly as possible. It gives them the freedom to say whatever they want during their laboring process but also allows for the birth team to take them seriously when and if they make that request.

on Creating Birth Preferences

by Samantha Huggins, *childbirth educator and co-director of Carriage House Birth*

I see writing your birth preferences as a two-part exercise in self-love. It's an opportunity to spoil yourself on paper. If you could have everything you wanted in a birth experience, exactly, no holds barred, what would it be? And then part two, if you needed intervention/management, what would your top ten bullets look like? Now for my favorite part: once you have completed this perfect ideal birth preferences list, go ahead and light that document on fire. That's not to say that you won't get your wishes—you deserve your ideal birth!—but you must be flexible. Your birth preferences list is a thread in the fabric of this particular birth story. From this single thread, you can now make choices for yourself, and your birth team will have a sense of what you are after and how to help guide you back to center by reminding you of what you had identified to begin with.

Monitoring the baby while in labor looks different depending on where you are giving birth. In a home birth or birthing center setting, a handheld Doppler ultrasound device is used to monitor the baby's heartbeat at regular intervals. The laboring person can move freely while being monitored. In a hospital setting, the external fetal heart rate monitor is primarily used to monitor the baby's well-being. Many hospitals will require you to have continuous fetal monitoring, and others require intermittent monitoring. Continuous monitoring will limit your mobility, so consider bringing a yoga ball to sit on (see page 104 to learn why). Some hospitals have wireless monitors, but unfortunately, they are not used universally.

Hep-lock

A hep-lock is an IV catheter that is placed in the vein, flushed with saline, and then capped off for potential later use.

Squat Bar

Sometimes referred to as a birthing bar, the squat bar can be attached to the labor bed to facilitate a squatting position. Gravity and the opening of the pelvis can help aid the pushing process.

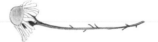

In a home birth or birthing center setting, you will be hydrating yourself orally with your favorite liquids. Only if it becomes medically necessary will your midwife or OB put in an IV. In some hospitals, it is standard practice to place an IV. It is done as a precaution to prevent dehydration. It also gives care providers immediate access to your veins should an emergency arise. You can request a hep-lock (saline lock) if you would like to move about freely and are planning on laboring without interventions. You can also request to not have an IV at all. You should know what your hospital's policy is on this to see what kind of pushback you may get. As long as you are not high risk, your body, your choice.

Using interventions during labor can vary depending on how your labor unfolds. Some care providers have a completely hands-off approach and don't intervene with the birthing process unless it becomes medically necessary. I wish more care providers took this approach. In 2017, the American Congress of Obstetricians and Gynecologists put out a study on approaches to limit intervention during labor and birth. If a person is having a healthy pregnancy and is deemed low risk, a hands-off approach with minimal interventions is suggested. It states that

Intervention During Labor

Intervention during labor is defined as an action by a care provider intervening or assisting in the laboring or birthing process. Common interventions are rupturing of the water (amniotomy), using Pitocin to speed labor, inductions, epidurals, continuous fetal monitoring, episiotomies, and cesarean birth. Be mindful that not all interventions are medically necessary. Many care providers schedule inductions due to time management or a heavy client load. Be sure to ask questions and express your feelings surrounding common interventions on your birth preferences document.

continuous one-to-one emotional support during labor is associated with improved outcomes and less need for interventions. Shout out to the badass birth partners, nurses, and birth doulas out there. *Woop woop!*

How do you envision pushing out your baby? Do you think you will respond well to being coached during pushing, or would you rather listen to your body's cues? I've witnessed babies coming out in almost every position imaginable. Different things work for different folks. Note that if you utilize an epidural, your options will become limited to the hospital bed.

Have you heard the term *delayed cord clamping*? This is when the umbilical cord is not cut until the cord stops pulsing. Research has found that when care providers delay clamping the cord for three minutes, the baby receives higher levels of iron, which helps prevent anemia. You can request in your birth preferences to delay the cord clamping. Most hospitals wait a few minutes until the cord stops pulsing. In a home birth setting, you can wait as long as you like.

Whatever way your little one enters the world, via vaginal or cesarean birth, if your baby is healthy and breathing well, you can request (demand) skin-to-skin contact. This request is honored most of the time if your baby is born vaginally. More and more hospitals are also honoring this request for surgical deliveries, because it is still very much a birth and

Lotus Birth

Lotus birth, or umbilical nonseverance, means the family waits for the cord to detach from their baby naturally rather than cutting it right after childbirth.

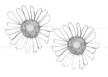

Skin-to-Skin Contact

Some of the benefits of skin-to-skin contact for newborns are keeping their body temperature stable, regulating their blood sugar, helping with the initiation of breastfeeding, calming them, and promoting bonding.

Vitamin K Shot

In newborns, adequate vitamin K levels are needed to prevent vitamin K deficiency bleeding (VKDB), a rare but life-threatening condition that causes uncontrolled bleeding, sometimes into the brain. The shot is administered shortly after birth.

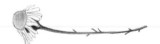

a sacred experience. Family-centered cesareans, also known as "gentle cesareans," are becoming more common due to informed consumer requests for them. If you don't want to or are unable to do skin-to-skin contact, your partner can. I tell partners to wear an easy-access top for slapping that baby right on their bare chest.

Newborn care procedures vary from state to state. You have more flexibility in declining or delaying these procedures in a home birth setting. In a hospital setting, I encourage all my clients to have an hour of uninterrupted skin-to-skin time before weighing, measuring, and

on Laboring

by Samantha Huggins, *childbirth educator and co-director of Carriage House Birth*

Thanks to media imagery and a culture steeped in fear of an ova-containing body and its power, it is very easy for us to sink our teeth into the fear, pain, and darkness surrounding a birth experience. We revel in negative stories about negative outcomes. Where does our connectedness to these narratives come from? Who do they really belong to? Your mother? Your grandmother? Your neighbor? A friend, sister, stranger? To sit down and meditate on our ideal birth experience is no small feat. It's an act of self-love that requires a certain quality of bravery. To do this, we must be able to overcome the negative narratives. It starts with the smallest step. It starts with hope. With hope, we receive possibility. If we have a thread of hope, we have a crack of light coming through the door. Open it. Daydream. Imagine peace. Imagine what you might do in the space between contractions. Will you sleep? Will you deeply exhale? Can you soften into this space? Can you use your power to honor relief?

administering shots. It is standard in most U.S. hospitals to administer erythromycin to the eyes to protect them from possible STD transmission. The vitamin K shot is also administered soon after birth. I had them wait until I established a latch with my wee one so I could soothe her at the breast immediately after. Some practices will offer the vitamin K orally, but this is less common. The baby will then be weighed, measured, and inked for footprints.

Circumcision is a huge debate in the United States. To cut or not to cut? My advice is to do your research. Watch a video of the procedure. Make an informed decision.

INFORMATION TO CONSIDER INCLUDING IN YOUR BIRTH PREFERENCES

- ○ Name
- ○ Partner (if applicable)
- ○ Estimated due date, scheduled induction, or surgical birth
- ○ Care provider
- ○ Place of delivery
- ○ Support team
- ○ Plans for managing intensity
- ○ Monitoring preferences
- ○ If you want an IV/hep-lock
- ○ Preferences for interventions
- ○ Pushing options
- ○ If you want delayed cord clamping
- ○ Preferences for skin-to-skin contact
- ○ Newborn procedures
- ○ Plan for infant feeding
- ○ Requests if a medically indicated induction becomes necessary
- ○ Requests if a surgical delivery becomes necessary (Can a doula attend? Would you prefer clear drapes? See page 126.)
- ○ If you'd prefer your hands not be bound (It is standard in many hospitals to put Velcro straps on your forearms as a precautionary measure in case you have an adverse reaction to the anesthesia.)
- ○ Requests if a transfer from home birth to hospital becomes necessary

Different things work for different folks.

WORKING THROUGH PAST TRAUMAS

Trigger warning: This section addresses sexual assault.

Before my first pregnancy, I had no idea that the sexual assault from my past could resurface and cause a traumatic childbirth experience. I thought that I had prepared myself thoroughly by reading all the Ina May Gaskin books, watching childbirth documentaries and videos, taking a childbirth education series with my partner, hiring a fantastic doula, and reviewing a ton of studies so I would know my choices and receive evidence-based care. I tucked my ugly trauma deep down and really believed that it would not impact the beautiful journey on which I was about to embark. I trusted in my body's ability to give birth. People are born every single day. We were all born from someone. I found comfort in knowing that I wasn't alone. Looking back, I realize that I greatly mini-mized how intense childbirth could be both physically and emotionally.

I was raped by a stranger when I was twenty-three years old. While I was being raped, I disassociated from my body. I watched myself being attacked from the ceiling. It was how I survived. I received support by attending therapy and trained as a rape crisis counselor to help advocate in the emergency room for other rape survivors. I actively worked on trying to heal my PTSD and anxiety. A couple of years later, I became pregnant with my first child. I never thought that there would be a link between giving birth and being raped.

My pregnancy was uncomplicated and, dare I say, easy. I was hoping and praying that the birth would unfold in the same way. When my due date came and went, I found myself getting extremely anxious. The fear of the unknown and the lack of control were triggering my PTSD big time. I (stupidly) took matters into my own hands and decided to gulp down a bunch of castor oil. I didn't consult my care provider or my birth team. My online research had me thinking I was an expert, and I had read that castor oil can stimulate the bowels, which can trigger contractions to start. I drank a bunch and nothing happened. A few hours later, I drank some more. Nothing. Defeated, I went to bed. (*Disclaimer*: Always consult with your care provider before trying *any* and *all* natural induction methods. You can put yourself and/or your baby in danger.)

I woke up a few hours later with severe diarrhea and ran to the bathroom. I was pooping my brains out when I realized that my contractions had started fast and furious, every three minutes. We drove to the hospital as I puked out the window the entire way. The labor was also fast and furious. I remember feeling like I was losing control of my body. It felt like I was being attacked. I once again disassociated from my physical body. I remember my birth from the ceiling of the hospital room. It was as if I were only a spectator at one of my major, life-altering events.

The feeling of not having control over what was happening to my body had triggered anxiety stemming from my sexual assault. If only I had acknowledged that the trauma from my past could potentially bubble to the surface, I may have had an easier childbirth. My heavy denial was clouding my ability to surrender and go along for the ride. I fought each contraction and tried to escape out of my body. When I pushed my daughter out, I felt like I was splitting in two or might die. I didn't. I was left feeling shocked and removed from the entire process.

My love for my newborn daughter is what healed me. She forced me to look at my trauma and move through it instead of tucking it away and hiding from it. My daughter taught me that I am a powerful human being capable of growing, birthing, and nurturing new life. I was able to evolve from being a victim to being a survivor.

If you have survived any type of sexual abuse or trauma, my advice is to acknowledge the darkness prior to childbirth and move through it. The way you move through it is up to you. Some people find comfort in talking to their support team, while others may find healing in quiet meditation. Please don't hesitate to seek out professional help. Know that you are *not* alone and there is loving protective light all around you.

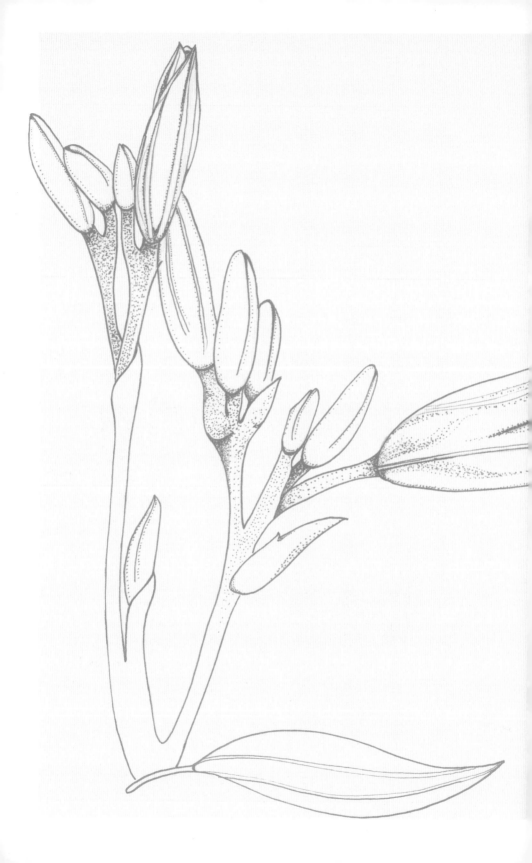

Part Two

Laboring and Birthing

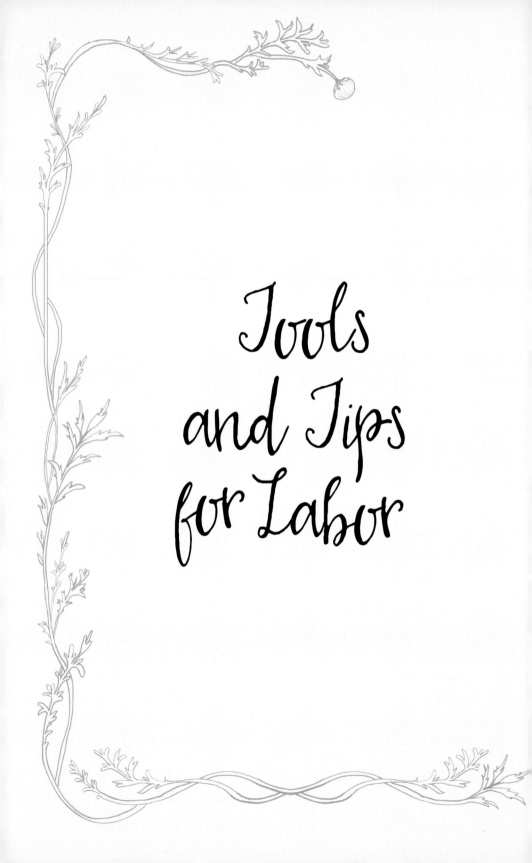

Tools
and Tips
for Labor

THE DAY YOU HAVE BEEN WAITING FOR HAS ARRIVED! THE beginning of your labor can be an extremely exciting and nerve-racking experience. Maybe for some, it's a day you've been dreading in whole or in part. Unless you are having a scheduled surgical delivery, you will experience the process of going into labor. There are many tools and tips that can aid you in this process. *Your positive mind-set is your biggest tool.* You can choose for your birth to be a positive experience regardless of how it unfolds. You hold that power. Please don't forget that. Now on to the other tools.

TOOLS FOR LABORING

Candles

Setting the mood is super important. If you are birthing at home, you can use good old-fashioned candles. If you are birthing in a hospital or birthing center, you will need to purchase battery-operated candles. Dimming the lights and setting the mood can greatly reduce anxiety.

Lip Balm

During labor, there can be lots of moaning, panting, and heavy breathing. This can lead to extremely dry and chapped lips. You definitely don't need chapped lips while trying to spring a human being from your body. Bring lip balm. Keep it nearby and have your partner or doula reapply it.

Essential Oils

I love using my essential oil diffuser regularly at home. Why not bring it along if you are birthing in a hospital or birthing center? Lavender is great for creating a calm and fresh atmosphere. My favorite essential oil birth blend is lavender, clary sage, and frankincense. I often use peppermint oil for energy, nausea, and aches and pains during labor. If you don't want to lug your diffuser in your hospital bag, you can purchase small nasal inhalers that you can keep in your pocket or handbag. These are great for surgical deliveries too, because the smell of the operating room can trigger anxiety and fear for some. During pregnancy, you can use aromatherapy to associate positive feelings with a particular smell. Any time you are joyful or feeling really good, take a whiff of lavender. Fast-forward to when you're in labor, and the smell of lavender will help trigger those feelings of joy.

Hair Bands
If you have long locks, bring your hair bands to keep all that hair out of your face. Better yet, braid your hair if it's long enough.

Hand Fan
A hand fan is great tool for cooling off a laboring person. You can appoint your birth partner to fanning duty, especially during the pushing phase when things seem to really heat up. My favorite fan is the small foldable paper kind.

Heating Pad
A heating pad can be used in early labor when the contractions feel like menstrual cramps. The consistent heat on your lower belly can be helpful in finding some relief. Heat can be used on the lower back to help ease back labor.

Laborade
For keeping hydrated. Make it ahead of time, perhaps in early labor. For a home birth, keep a pitcher in the fridge. For a hospital delivery, consider storing it in a large water bottle and bringing it with you.

⅓ cup (80 ml) fresh lemon juice
⅓ cup (80 ml) honey
¼ tsp salt
¼ tsp baking soda
1 or 2 calcium magnesium tablets, crushed

Combine all ingredients and add enough water to make 1 quart (1 L). Serve cold.

Massage Oil

You might be someone who doesn't want to be touched at all during your labor, or you may want *all* the touching and the massaging during your birth. Either way, it's a good idea to have a nice massage oil on hand. I typically suggest an odorless massage oil or an arnica massage oil. Arnica can help soothe sore muscles and ease pain. It's perfect for laboring bodies.

Pillows

Hospitals always seem to be out of pillows. If you are having a hospital or a birthing center birth, bring an extra pillow or two from home. Make sure you put on a pillowcase that's a pattern or bright color so you don't mix it up with the hospital's pillows. As silly as it sounds, this can be a game changer. Comfort during and after childbirth is important.

Snacks

Labor can sometimes be long and hard. You can't run a marathon on an empty tank. Bring snacks for yourself and your birth team. Due to the risk of vomiting during labor, it's best to avoid foods with high acidity. Stick to broth, yogurt, applesauce, fruit (watermelon is a top choice), smoothies, bananas with almond butter, and Popsicles. If you don't feel like eating during labor, that's okay. You'll be starving after giving birth, so the snacks won't go to waste. Also, make sure you know the rules on snacking while laboring at the hospital or birthing center. Some facilities only allow clear liquids and ice chips for laboring folks. Research suggests that it is perfectly safe to eat during labor.

Talisman

Having a talisman to hold in your palm during labor can have a very calming and powerful effect. Many people choose various objects for different reasons. I chose a large chuck of rose quartz during my last pregnancy. It felt like I was holding a piece of love in my hand. It gave me a focal point in a very intense labor. Smooth stones can be a nice option to hold. The pressure of the object in your palm can serve as a distraction from the intense labor waves. Pick an object that has some emotional value.

When I attend a birth as the doula, I will often bring a special rock for my laboring client to hold. I charge the rock beforehand with my positive energy and love. I typically pick rose quartz for love, emotional balance, and peace. I also love to bring polished malachite, which is known as the *midwife stone* as it is said to stimulate contractions, ease labor intensity, and protect the laboring person and baby.

Washcloth

A washcloth can be heated up or dipped in a bucket of ice water. Warm compresses may feel really nice on your lower back during contractions. A cold washcloth is ideal for the transition phase of labor and during pushing. I vividly remember my midwife pressing a cool washcloth on my forehead minutes before I pushed out my last baby.

Water Bottle

A water bottle with a bendy straw is a must-have labor essential because it's your job to hydrate. Take a sip after every contraction. The bendy straw is important too, because it's easy to sip from it in any position, even lying down.

Yoga Ball

One of your pregnancy/laboring must-haves is a yoga ball. It is often called a *birth ball* by doulas and birth workers. During my pregnancy, I swapped out my office desk chair for a yoga ball. It helped strengthen my lower back and supported my pelvis. The use of a yoga ball during pregnancy can help encourage optimal fetal positioning. During labor, it can be helpful to bounce on during contractions, and it can even accelerate your labor. Sitting on the ball and drawing figure eights with your hips can help bring your baby down and out. You can utilize the ball for support while kneeling and leaning forward. Rocking back and forth while leaning on the ball may be a labor rhythm that works for you. In a hospital birth setting, you may need to be monitored frequently, which will require you being tethered to the external fetal monitor. Many hospitals do not have wireless monitors. The yoga ball will allow you to be up and out of the bed while being monitored. This can be especially helpful for an induction in which you may need to be monitored for the entire laboring process. If you end up not using the birth ball during the laboring process, you can use it after you give birth to soothe a cranky newborn. Snuggle and bounce.

Yoga Mat

A yoga mat is great for laboring in many different positions. I folded mine up and knelt on it while in the shower. The yoga mat makes it much easier on the knees. I've also seen many partners grab a quick snooze on the hospital floor if a pull-out chair or extra bed is not available.

Crystals

I believe in the power of crystals. Crystals come from the earth and can help you tap into your own healing energy. I feel relaxed and balanced when I incorporate crystals into my everyday life. Whether they are really magic or it's simply just the power of suggestion, I'm sold. I used a small polished worry stone to rub whenever I got anxious during my pregnancy and birth.

TIPS FOR LABORING

Breathing

Please don't forget to breathe. When we become tense, we forget to breathe. Without breath, the contractions can become painful and overwhelming. Try to breathe fully and rhythmically during your surges. You don't need to learn any fancy breathing techniques (unless you want to); just remember to breathe. Your breath is a guide through the contractions. Focus on your breath as soon as you feel a surge building. Keep following your breath by focusing on the inhales and exhales until you are at the other end of the surge.

Contraction Timer

Download a contraction timer app. Only start timing your contractions if you notice a pattern starting to develop or the surges start building in intensity. Don't become too obsessed with the damn timer app, though. Put it down occasionally and find your flow. Your care provider or doula may ask what your labor pattern looks like. This helps them figure out where you may be in the laboring process. Timing labor contractions may be a great task for your labor partner or birth doula. The busier you become in labor the less likely you will want to time your own contractions.

For folks who are trying to avoid an epidural and/or other potential interventions, staying home until a strong labor pattern unfolds is ideal. Aim for 3-1-1 or 5-1-1. What the heck does that mean? Contractions or surges are 5 minutes apart for a minute long and for the duration of 1 hour: 5-1-1. Your labor pattern can indicate how far along you may be in the laboring process. Also, 5-1-1 suggests you may be in active labor, or around 5 centimeters dilated. And 3-1-1 may mean that you are much further along in the process and closer to the transition phase of labor. Don't be disappointed if your cervix doesn't follow this rule. Your cervix is *not* a crystal ball.

When to Head to the Hospital

Many of my laboring clients wonder about the best time to head to the hospital. I first suggest that they check in with their care providers to see what their suggestions are. If they are safe to stay at home for a little while, I suggest hopping in the shower. If the warm water slows down labor, we know that we still have some time. If the contractions remain the same or start to intensify, we know things are picking up. I once had a client hop in the shower, and as soon as she relaxed in the warm water she started bearing down (pushing). We hightailed it to the hospital, where she pushed her baby out within minutes.

Hip Squeeze

The hip squeeze pushes the hips into a relaxed position, relieving the pressure from the contractions. Have your birth partner and/or doula learn the double hip squeeze, as it can be an extremely effective comfort measure while laboring.

Here's how to do it: The laboring person is standing or leaning forward, on hands and knees, laying facedown over a birth ball, or sitting on a birth ball. The idea is to have full access to the lower back to be able to apply pressure to the hips.

Place your hands on your partner's hip bones. Move your palms down a bit lower into the divots just below the hip bones.

Apply counter pressure during the duration of a contraction. Keep your elbows out while pushing in. Listen to the laboring person's cues as to where and how hard to be pressing.

Hydrotherapy

Consider using a shower or tub to help manage the intensity of your labor. Some folks even refer to the bathtub as nature's epidural. Be sure to ask if your labor and deliver floor has a working shower or tub if that's something you are interested in.

Birthing Atmosphere

The birthing atmosphere/vibe is extremely important. When you give birth in a hospital, it is hard to claim that space as your own. One of my clients had an induction planned and decided to go all out decorating her hospital room before she started. She had banners hanging on the wall with positive affirmations, soft music playing, photographs of loved ones, and an aromatherapy diffuser. I felt like I had just stepped into a luxury spa. She provided goodies for the hospital staff and every person that walked into the room left with a smile. She had a wonderful birth. I believe the energy that she put into creating her sacred birthing space was the reason it was so wonderful.

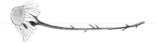

Labor Art/Birth Altar

Bring photographs or inspiring birth art to a hospital or birthing center birth. Claim the birthing space as your own. This can greatly reduce anxiety and fear. Creating a birth altar during pregnancy will provide a focal point for your labor. You can fill it with personal objects that make you feel empowered and supported. For example, my birthing altars included pink roses, huge chunks of rose quartz and tourmaline, an Aztec birthing statue, a strand of beads filled with the love and intentions of my closest girlfriends, a birth art painting, a vagina necklace, and a few birth affirmation cards. My favorite birth affirmation card read, "The contractions cannot be stronger than you, because they are you."

Music

Does music play a part in your life? If so, I strongly suggest making a labor playlist. I've attended births during which the clients danced their baby into the world with Bob Marley. I've witnessed a birth with Metallica's *Ride the Lightning* playing as the birth soundtrack. The sounds of nature may do the trick for you. Who knows? Music is a wonderful tool for setting the mood and claiming the birthing space as your own. I strongly recommend to all the cesarean birthers to make a playlist as well for when you are in the operating room. Keep one earbud in while they are prepping for the birth. Choose music that calms you or makes you feel powerful.

Pee

Please remember to pee during your labor. The baby will have more room to move down and out when your bladder is empty. A full bladder can halt the laboring process. As the baby descends, it can sometimes be hard to feel the urge to pee. If you are having difficulty peeing, you can try putting a few drops of peppermint oil in the toilet water. It has been known to help aid the process. I once supported a client in labor who was having a hard time emptying her bladder. The nurse suggested using a straight catheter to empty the bladder. Because my client was laboring without an epidural, this would have proven very uncomfortable. I put five drops of peppermint oil in the toilet and had her try again. *Success*! The smell of peppermint oil can sometimes help release the bladder.

Visualization

Many birth doula clients of mine like to utilize guided visualization and meditation during their labor. There are many options that you can download and play. You can also have your partner or doula guide you through a visualization. I always tend to lean toward being on a beautiful beach with the sun warming my skin and the ocean waves are crashing and spaying a cool mist on my body . . . you get the gist! My cervix is a flower blooming. My contractions are waves rising and falling. Using visualization techniques in labor can reduce fear and release tension.

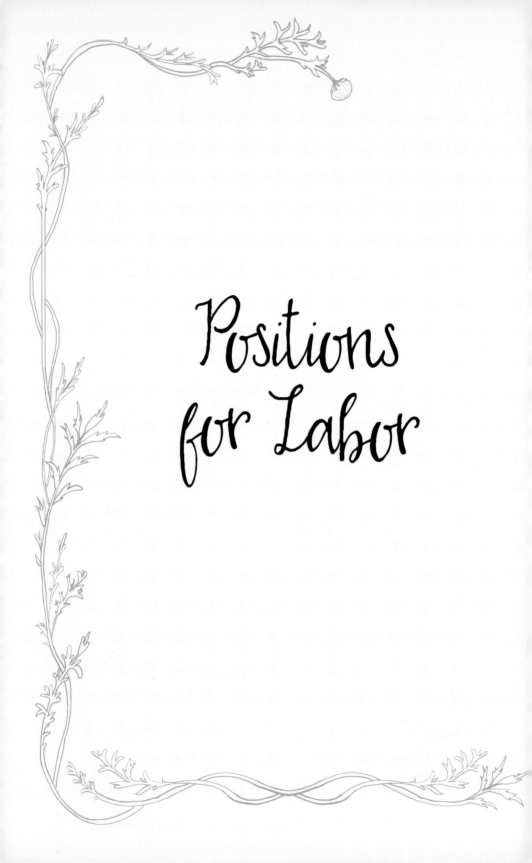

Positions for Labor

DURING YOUR LABOR, CHANGING POSITIONS OFFERS
several benefits. Being upright and changing your position can help
encourage the baby to descend into the birth canal. This can also speed
your labor. Movement can also be a wonderful tool for managing labor
intensity. Taking a childbirth education class will teach you some ideal
laboring positions. Break out that birth ball and get creative. Here are a
few positions to try and why.

Hands and knees: This position is ideal for relieving back pressure and/
or back labor. If a baby is posterior (sunny-side up), the hands and knees
position can help encourage your little one to move into an optimal
position. Pelvic rocking while in the hands and knees position can help
the baby move down the pelvis.

Lunges: Lunges are another great way to encourage a posterior baby to
rotate into an anterior position. Prop your leg up on a chair and lunge
toward your knee, with your knee facing out. This technique will widen
the pelvis, allowing for the babe to rotate.

Squatting: Squatting during labor is said to greatly reduce your overall
time in labor. The average first-timer typically has a longer labor (twelve
to twenty-four hours). Squatting widens the pelvis and utilizes gravity
to help that baby move down and out. This position can help dilate
your cervix. The only downside is that it can be downright tiring for the
ankles, knees, and hips.

Side lying: Side lying can be a wonderful position in which to get some
rest in between contractions. If you end up utilizing relief in the form
of an epidural, flipping from side to side is super helpful in continuing
to encourage the baby to descend. This is a great time to introduce the
peanut ball (see page 114). Putting a peanut ball between your legs in
a side-lying position can open your pelvic outlet considerably. This is a
wonderful tool to incorporate if an epidural is introduced or if you are
required to labor in bed.

Posterior vs. Anterior

A posterior position (occiput posterior, or OP) means that the babe is facing up, or "sunny-side up," instead of facedown (optimal), so the hardest part of babe's head rests near your lower back instead of your belly. This position often results in a longer labor, because the head has to rotate further during labor in order to be born.

Anterior (occiput anterior, or OA) position is when the baby's head is facing down and the back of the baby's head is toward the front of the pregnant person. This is the ideal position for baby.

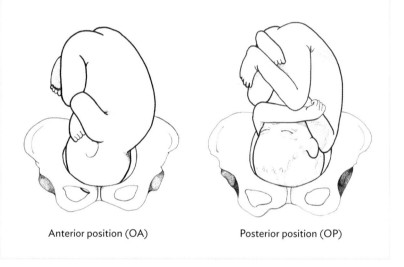

Anterior position (OA)   Posterior position (OP)

Sitting on the toilet: This happens to be my favorite spot for laboring. Light some candles and turn off the lights in the bathroom. We are taught at an early age to hold in our urine, bowel movements, and farts. We are constantly holding. Sitting on the toilet is the one place we really release everything and stop holding. Your pelvic floor releases and your baby will descend much easier in this position.

Slow dancing: Do you remember, during the eighth grade dance, slow dancing to "Stairway to Heaven"? Well, I do. The slow dance is also a great laboring position. The swaying movement helps keep your hips moving and encourages the baby to rotate down and out. Throw on your birthing jams and get to dancing that baby out.

Walking: Walking is a great way to power through your labor. Gravity helps the baby descend. Walking can also kick your early labor into high gear. If you have steps in your home or apartment, you can walk up and down to really move things along. Make sure you listen to your body and rest when you start to feel fatigued. Don't overdo it.

SIMPLE AFFIRMATIONS FOR CHILDBIRTH

"I can."
"I am enough."
"I will birth my baby."
"I am fierce."
"I am love."
"I am light."
"This is good intensity."
"I am riding the wave."
"Eyes on the prize."
"My ancestors are guiding me."
"I am laboring with purpose."
"I am birthing with grace."
"I am easing my baby into the world."
"Each contraction brings me closer to meeting my baby."
"I am filled with abundance and love."
"I am not alone."
"Love is guiding me."

Peanut Ball

The peanut ball is an oblong exercise ball that is shaped like a large peanut. It is being used in some hospitals to help decrease cesarean rates, mostly when a laboring person needs to remain in bed. The ball is placed between the legs to widen the pelvic outlet. This is a wonderful tool for clients who have an epidural and want to promote dilation and descent.

INDUCTIONS

Labor induction is the use of medication or other methods to bring on labor. Essentially, you are tricking the body into labor. Why, you may ask? Sometimes it is medically necessary to induce for the safety of the baby and the laboring person. An elective induction can be attempted after 39 weeks. The emotional well-being of the pregnant person can also be a factor in deciding when to induce. Your care provider's vacation plans, however, should not be a factor in deciding when and if you should induce. Just saying. With all that said, please be aware that your chance of a surgical delivery increases if you are a first-timer and if your cervix is not favorable for induction.

The one myth that I would like to dispel is that setting up an induction is an easier route through labor. I can't tell you how many of my clients who elected to get induced later regretted their decision. If you are going to have an elective induction, that's fine, just know what it entails so you can make an informed decision. You don't just pop in and quickly have a baby; it's usually quite a process that can range on average from four to forty-eight hours. Some folks won't have a choice in the matter at all, because they are being induced for medical reasons. You may, however, have some say in the methods your care provider is using for inducing.

Bishop Score

Published in 1964 by Edward Bishop, the Bishop score is a vaginal examine that determines how favorable your cervix is to being induced. The score ranges from 0 to 12. The higher the score, the better chances of a vaginal delivery.

Possible Reasons for Induction

- You've gone past your due date. Most practices in the United States are comfortable with you going until forty-two weeks of pregnancy. After that point, induction is often strongly encouraged. With twins, thirty-eight weeks is suggested. (I personally carried my twins safely until forty weeks with extra scans and monitoring.)

- You have a condition in which the baby is safer being born than having you remain pregnant. These conditions could include diabetes, preeclampsia, high blood pressure, fetal growth restrictions, and infections.

- Your water has ruptured and active labor has not started. You will have a discussion with your care provider to determine how long it is okay to wait until active labor starts. Some practices have you come in immediately, while others have you wait until up to twenty-four hours.

Methods of Induction

There are several methods used for the induction of labor. Your cervix will probably determine which approach your care provider will choose. If your cervix is closed and not ripe, it will more than likely be a cervical ripening agent. They are used to soften and efface (thin) the cervix. Cervadil and Cytotec are the most commonly used cervical ripeners in the United States. One of these medications is placed in the vagina in the hopes of preparing the cervix for labor. It stays in for up to twelve hours and is then removed. It may be removed even sooner if and when contractions start. Sometimes another dose is required. Many times, care providers suggest starting this process in the evening so you can sleep through this part. There can be a lot of waiting until things really get moving.

If your cervix is ripe (soft) and dilated (open) already, sometimes a membrane sweep can do the trick. A membrane sweep, or stripping of the membranes, is when your care provider inserts a finger in your cervix and moves it a circular motion, separating the amniotic sac from the cervix. It doesn't feel particularly good either. *Ouch!* It can produce prostaglandins, which may kick-start your labor. If you are dilated enough, your care provider may also suggest breaking your water to get things moving.

A Foley balloon catheter is a tool for dilating the cervix manually without the use of medications. The catheter is placed between the lower part of the uterus and the amniotic sac. It is then filled with saline (like a balloon) to create pressure on the cervix. The balloon will eventually fall out and the cervix will dilate. Labor may start from the Foley, or Pitocin may be introduced now that the cervix is more favorable for labor. This Foley balloon is not extremely common nowadays, but it can be effective. Ask your care provider if this may be an option for you. I've had doula clients find this procedure mildly uncomfortable and others find it unbearable. Our bodies process these interventions very differently.

Pitocin is used for the induction of labor in a hospital setting. Care providers use Pitocin to start contractions and to strengthen them. Your

Cervix Softness

My midwife explained to me that a cervix during pregnancy is firm like the tip of your nose. When labor begins, the cervix starts to soften and can be compared to a pair of pouty lips. That's a ripe cervix. Great visual, huh!?

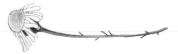

Oxytocin

Also known as the *love hormone*, oxytocin is a hormone released by the pituitary gland that causes increased contraction of the uterus during labor and stimulates the ejection of milk into the ducts of the breasts.

body naturally produces oxytocin, which creates contractions. Pitocin is an amped-up synthetic version of oxytocin. It is administered via an IV in your arm and is periodically increased to get a desired effect. The contractions should be long enough and strong enough to create cervical change (around two to three minutes apart). The amount of Pitocin needed varies from person to person. I've encountered clients who only need a whiff of Pitocin while others are at the maximum suggested dose. Your cervix should be "favorable," or ripe, to start an induction with straight Pitocin. Pitocin doesn't create dilation of the cervix; it creates the contractions that cause the cervix to dilate. There are risks associated with using Pitocin, and I would encourage you to do your research and discuss your options with your care provider.

Please remember to eat a hearty meal before heading into an induction. You never know how long it will be before you have a chance to eat again. Many hospitals have an ice chips–only rule for all laboring people having a labor induction.

Empowered Induction

One of my favorite births that I've attended was an unexpected induction. My client had her heart set on the birthing center but ended up risking out and needing to be induced on the regular labor and delivery floor. She was disappointed, but focused on having an amazing birthing experience. She opted to labor without using an epidural. Swaying her hips, using the birthing ball, and having a supportive partner got her through. She delivered while standing up. It was magnificent.

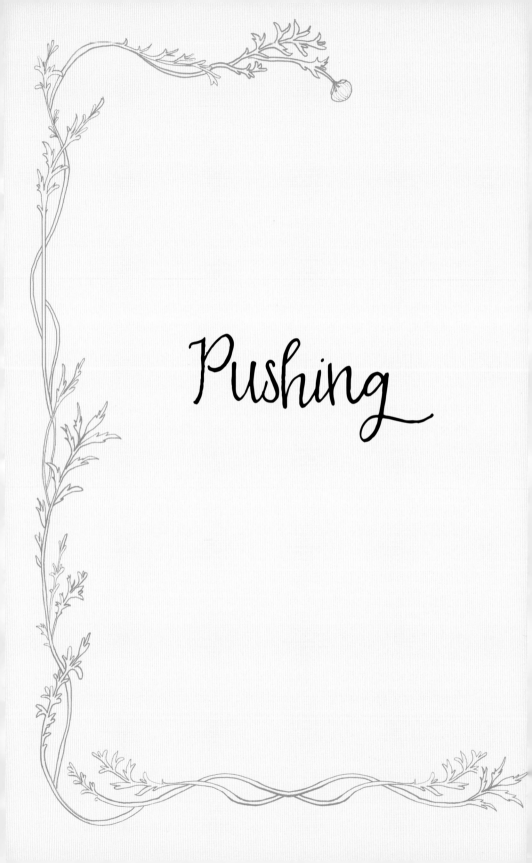

Pushing

ALL RIGHT, YOU ARE FULLY DILATED (10 CM), AND IT'S time to push out your baby. Now what? Pushing can take anywhere from thirty minutes up to three hours for a first-timer. Again, this is just an average range. It could be as short as a few minutes or as long as several hours. I can't tell you how many of my doula clients believe that once they reach 10 cm, a baby just pops out. That does happen sometimes, but more often than not there's some real hard work that needs to be put in to get the baby to come down and out. Be easy on yourself. Pushing is on-the-job training.

Waiting until you have an actual urge to push will help guide you in getting your baby out. Many folks are shocked by how similar the feeling of pressure in their bottom is to taking a massive poop. We are taught at an early age to hold our bowels and our urine, so releasing our pelvic floor and allowing a baby to come out can feel counterintuitive and be very challenging. And let's get real: you might poop. Most people do. If you're pushing in the right place, the chances are pretty high that you're going to poop.

The pushing phase will be very drastically different depending on whether you utilize relief from an epidural or not. Here's what to expect.

PUSHING WITHOUT AN EPIDURAL

When you are laboring unmedicated, it is much easier to feel the urge to push. Your body guides you. You will push with each surge that you get. Rest in between. Trust your intuition. You are also given the freedom to decide which position feels best to push in. Standing, squatting, lying down, or in the tub are all options available to you.

Spontaneous pushing, or fetal ejection reflex, is when your body takes over and uncontrollably expels the baby. There is no pushing effort needed. This happened with two of my births, and let me just tell you, they were the most intense and surreal experiences of my life. It is rare to see spontaneous pushing in a hospital setting. Most hospital births are medically managed and not undisturbed. As a doula, I've witnessed a handful of home births during which the client had the fetal ejection reflex. In each, the environment was quiet, calm, and dimly lit. The laboring person had a surge of energy and then a large contraction that ejected the baby without the need for pushing. Physiological birth is, unfortunately, rarely seen in our current highly medicalized climate.

PUSHING WITH AN EPIDURAL

When you have an epidural, it is much harder to feel some of the sensations required to help you push out a baby. Waiting to labor down or feel the urge to push can be extremely helpful, and this is usually felt as pressure after an epidural. Laboring down is when you are fully dilated (10 cm) and wait an hour or more to begin pushing. Guided pushing is often utilized for clients who have decided to get the epidural. Your care provider will instruct you to push for three intervals per contraction, which can also be utilized in non-epidural births. Tuck your chin to your chest. Hold your breath like you are diving under water and push like you are pooping. This is when your nurse or care provider may start chanting, "*Push!*" This approach may or may not work for you.

For many laboring people, the ability to move freely helps them manage the intensity of the contractions. Being forced to stay still and be constantly monitored can be quite a challenge.

You will be somewhat limited in positions because of the epidural. The most common position for pushing with an epidural is in a semi-reclined position in the hospital bed. You can also try pushing on your side, or perhaps you have enough strength to try a hands and knees position. I have been a part of epidural-assisted births in which we've been able to utilize the squat bar and positioned the bed in a throne-like position to take advantage of gravity.

If you become too numb from the epidural and have difficulty pushing, your care provider can turn down or turn off the epidural

Orgasmic Birth

Orgasmic birth is a concept promoted by longtime birth doula trainer and childbirth educator Debra Pascali-Bonaro. The idea arose from her many years of witnessing births that were empowering and even pleasurable. She defines orgasmic birth as "broad enough to include those who describe birth as ecstatic and specific enough to give voice to those who actually feel the contractions of orgasm and climax at the moment of delivery."

Pushing in the Mirror

Consider using a mirror while pushing. It can be very helpful to physically see the progress you are making.

medication. You will begin to have more sensation and can use the contractions as momentum to help move your baby down and out.

Don't get discouraged while pushing. Epidural or not, the rule "two steps forward, one step back" often applies. Babies rock and roll a bit before they come under the pubic bone. Once they are under, it's called crowning. The burning and stretching during crowning is called the *ring of fire*, just like the Johnny Cash song. Don't worry, it doesn't last long. This is stretching your vagina to prevent tearing.

VAGINAL BIRTH

Now here comes your baby, *bloop! Sweet relief!* The sense of physical relief that follows is indescribable. The only thing that ruins it is having to push out your placenta. Don't worry, though, it has no bones. The placenta arrives from a few minutes up to 30 minutes after baby is born. Your care

Fundal Massage

Fundal massage is done by firmly massaging the top of the uterus (the fundus) to reduce bleeding and cramping of the uterus after childbirth.

provider will make sure it's intact and give you a bit of a fundal massage once it's delivered. And FYI, it's not a massage that feels particularly good. Care providers do it to prevent bleeding post-delivery. Ask your care provider to show you the placenta as well. It's a fascinating organ that sustained life inside your body. You may not be planning on consuming or encapsulating your placenta, but please pay it some respect. Also, it is within your rights to request your placenta if you want it. Most hospitals have a waiver you can sign to release it. You can plant it in your yard, make a placenta smoothie, encapsulate your placenta by drying it into a powder and sealing it into capsules, or make placenta artwork prints.

Now that your placenta is delivered and examined, you will be assessed for tearing. *Eek.* I know this part sucks, but it is completely normal. The majority of first-timers will have some tearing. There are four degrees of tearing. A first-degree tear is the smallest of tears in the lining of the vagina, and the range goes up to a fourth-degree tear, which is a deep tear that goes through the muscles and the rectal lining. Thank goodness fourth-degree tearing is not very common. If necessary, your care provider will use stitches to put you back together again. This may take a bit of time and may not be particularly comfortable. Your care provider can use topical lidocaine if you didn't have an epidural to minimize discomfort while suturing. Most stitches will dissolve over time. Your wound will be quite tender as it heals. The discomfort can last several weeks, so take it easy. You don't want to bust a stitch.

Placenta Options

I am not a placenta pusher. If you are not interested in ingesting your placenta, then don't. There is currently not enough significant research on the possible benefits of placenta consumption. No pharmaceutical company will make money on placenta encapsulation, so they don't do much research on the potential benefits. Some of the possible benefits include a decreased risk of postpartum depression, increased milk supply, restoration of iron levels, increased energy, and increased oxytocin. I encapsulated my second set of twins' placenta (it was massive) and noticed a marked difference in my postpartum experience. I had far more energy and produced more milk. I am not sure if it was my "happy pills" or just a streak of good luck. Either way, I was okay with it, even if it was just a placebo effect.

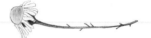

CESAREAN BIRTH

I will not refer to a cesarean delivery as a *C-section*. I prefer *C-birth* or *cesarean birth*. Meat is sectioned by a butcher; you birth your baby. The way we say things has a profound impact on how we view them. A cesarean birth is when an incision (around 6 inches [15cm]) is made to the lower abdomen and uterus to deliver a baby/babies surgically. Cesarean birth is still a birth. Don't let anyone tell you otherwise. It takes bravery to lay down your body to be cut open to deliver your baby safely into this world. That is courageous.

Still, the truth is that the cesarean birth rate in the United States is far too high. Around one in three expectant people will have a cesarean birth. It's the most common surgical procedure in the country. This high cesarean rate is not producing better birth outcomes. The maternal mortality rate has increased, *not* improved, in the last two decades. The infant mortality rate as of 2016 is 5.8 per 1,000 births. That's double the rate of countries such as Japan and Iceland. So what gives?

Experts suggest that many of the unnecessary cesareans being performed in the United States could be due to defensive medicine. The risk of being sued prevents care providers from practicing obstetrics. I recently had a long conversation with an extremely disheartened obstetrician about this very topic. She shared that many hospitals put extremely conservative parameters on childbirth, and healthy, low-risk patients are falling victim to unnecessary cesareans. It's becoming a huge conflict of interest for care providers, who are being forced to practice in constant fear of being sued. To reiterate, this is just anecdotal evidence. Other suspected reasons are failed elective inductions and scheduling conflicts with care providers.

Let me be clear: A necessary cesarean is a wonderful, lifesaving procedure. We should be grateful that cesarean births save lives. I also respect cesareans by choice. You never know why someone has decided to have a surgical delivery in a normal pregnancy. Past traumas and emotional well-being, for example, may be factors in deciding to have one.

Family-centered Cesarean

Have you heard the term *family-centered cesarean*? Also known as *gentle cesarean*, the term is pretty self-explanatory. It's a surgical delivery in which the family is the primary focus of the experience. The family will be able to express their concerns and wishes for the birth and have these requests honored by the medical team. Just because a baby is being born surgically does not mean that it has to be treated like a standard surgical procedure. The birth of a child should be treated like a sacred and monumental event.

Most hospitals and care providers are not on board with family-centered cesareans just yet. The requests for them have been growing rapidly, though. You are the consumer. You have the power to create positive change in your birthing experience. How's that for empowering?

on Gentle Cesareans

by Village Obstetrics, *obstetrician-gynecologist practice in New York City*

All cesareans should be gentle. Find out if your hospital/doctor has this philosophy.

Apgar Score

The Apgar score is a test used to determine how well the newborn baby handled the birthing process. The test also determines whether the newborn needs additional medical or emergency care. Apgar is an acronym for appearance, pulse, grimace, activity, and respiration.

I encourage you to read the questions below in case you are faced with a surgical birth. Things rarely goes as planned, and it is always best to be informed of all the potential birthing choices you may have. I often find that those of my doula clients who are the most afraid and unwilling to even consider a surgical delivery end up having a cesarean birth. Dive into where it's uncomfortable. Educate yourself on all the what-ifs. Remember that it is within your rights to know what the cesarean rate is at the hospital where you are delivering.

Here is a list of potential questions that you may want to ask your care provider before your planned surgical delivery. Please be aware that in the case of an emergency, a preterm delivery, or a baby at risk for a low

Apgar score, these requests will not be able to be facilitated. Your safety and your baby's safety will always come first. As they should.

- Can I avoid being strapped down for the surgery?
- May my whole support team (partner, doula, family member, etc.) be present for the delivery?
- May I have one of my support team members take photographs of the birth?
- Is a clear drape available, or can the drape be lowered so I can see my baby being born? Can the bed be raised a bit so I can see?
- Can the EKG electrodes be placed toward my back and side to leave my chest clear for skin-to-skin contact?
- Can the blood pressure cuff, IV, and oximeter be placed on my non-dominant arm?
- Can I get a nondrowsy anti-nausea medication, if possible?
- What type of medications does the anesthesiologist give during the surgery? Do I have the option of a medication or sedative that won't make me forget the birth?
- If possible, can the medical team avoid chatter that is unrelated to the birth? We understand that this may be a routine procedure for you, but for us this is the birth of our child!
- Can we bring in our own music and aromatherapy? (A nasal inhaler is perfect for the operating room.)
- Can delayed cord clamping be facilitated?
- Is skin-to-skin contact able to be facilitated if baby is doing well? Can the baby be suctioned on my chest?
- Can you show me the placenta after delivery?
- If the baby is healthy, will we be separated at any point? Can I room in with my baby?

CESAREAN AFFIRMATIONS

Here are a few cesarean affirmations that you can repeat to yourself during your birth. Affirmations can greatly reduce anxiety and fear before, during, and after a cesarean delivery.

"I am birthing my baby in a room filled with love."
"It's okay to be afraid."
"Cesarean birth is birth."
"My body is going to heal."
"I love my baby."
"It takes courage to birth my baby this way."
"I am surrendering to the flow of life."

Affirmations can greatly reduce anxiety and fear before, during, and after a cesarean delivery.

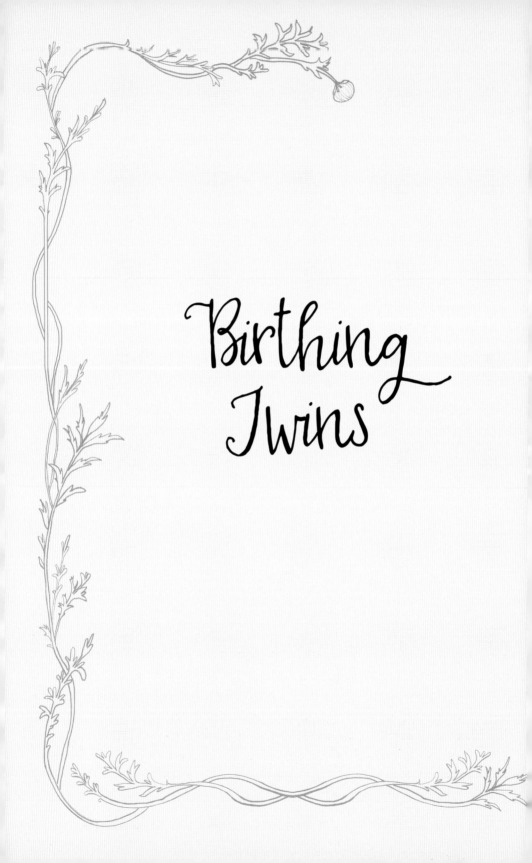

Birthing Twins

I AM EXTREMELY EXCITED TO INCLUDE A TWIN pregnancy/childbirth section in this book. When I was pregnant with my twins (both sets), I struggled to find positive and empowering information on twin pregnancy and childbirth. I found that most books taught you how to be a good patient and how to prepare for the worst-case scenarios. I'm all for being prepared, and I am well aware that things may not go as planned, but what about a healthy balance of information? I didn't hear any of the positive twin childbirth stories. Most of the information I found was not framed as choices. We are not being fully informed about what choices we do have.

The birth of my twin daughters (the first set of twins) inspired me to become a birth doula. I really liked my obstetrician, but I had no idea that she wouldn't be the one to deliver me. Many practices have five to eight doctors on rotation. She didn't mention this to me. She discouraged me from hiring a doula and strongly encouraged me to get an epidural (in hindsight these were red flags). While I was in labor, the on-call obstetrician offered me a cesarean casually because it would be an easier delivery for *him*. My babies were not in distress and were both head down. I declined the cesarean and birthed my twins vaginally without complications.

Not all twins can or should be born vaginally, but we deserve a right to try. Many care providers are not trained in breech deliveries and cannot deliver you vaginally unless your twins are both in a head-down position (vertex/vertex). There are, however, very skilled and well-trained obstetricians and midwives who can deliver twins vaginally if baby A is head down and baby B is breech. There are a few who will even deliver twins in a double breech presentation. Do your research and ask lots of questions. Finding a care provider who supports your birthing wishes is extremely important when you are pregnant with multiples.

I've been fortunate enough to assist numerous twin families on their childbearing journeys. I've supported gorgeous planned cesarean births and unmedicated vaginal twin births. One of my clients recently had a double vaginal breech delivery with her twins. Her care provider was skilled in breech birth, and the delivery was uncomplicated.

PREPARING FOR A TWIN BIRTH

I strongly encourage you to take a twin prep class as most childbirth classes focus on singleton pregnancies. A twin pregnancy is different. Here are a few questions to guide you on creating twin birth preferences.

- What type of atmosphere (dimmed lights, aromatherapy, music, etc.) will help you feel most comfortable?
- Will you be able to deliver vaginally with one breech or transverse-positioned twin? Or both breech?
- What is your care provider's view on cesarean births and when to perform one?
- When does your care provider recommend an induction in a twin pregnancy? At thirty-eight weeks? At forty-two weeks? What are your thoughts on inductions?
- Where will you deliver your twins? The operating room? A birth center? Home?
- Who (partner, doula, friend, family member, etc.) would you like present for the birth? How many staff or other personnel should you expect at the delivery?
- Do you plan on having an epidural or pain medication, or do you plan to avoid them?
- What is your care provider's view on delayed cord clamping?
- Are you planning on encapsulating your twins' placenta? What is the hospital's policy on releasing twin placentas?
- If you plan to deliver in the hospital, will your twins be able to room in with you after the delivery?
- What if your twins require a neonatal intensive care unit (NICU) stay? What are the hospital's policies?
- Do you plan on breastfeeding? If so, do you have access to a breast pump and/or lactation support?
- Do you have a postpartum support plan? A postpartum doula? Family?

TAKING TWINS HOME

Now that your twins have arrived, you will need to learn how to embrace chaos. Learn to surrender a bit to the process. Parenting newborn twins taught me that one of the babies will always need to wait while you tend to the other's needs. All the struggles are worth it for the rewards of having twins. Hang in there. I feel blessed that I have two sets of twins.

Below is a homecoming checklist for twins. Your lifestyle will play a role in deciding what items to obtain, so just use this list as guidance when preparing.

- Twins' daily schedule/logbook. This is not for everyone, but it can be very helpful if you have preemie twins and are keeping track of feedings and weight gain.
- 1–2 cribs or 2 bassinets. My twins shared a crib until they started rolling around and waking each other up. Some families choose to co-sleep. Research what option is best for your family and do it safely.
- 2 car seats
- Double stroller
- Wrap or carrier for babywearing
- 4–8 crib/bassinet sheets
- 6–10 receiving blankets
- 2–4 heavy blankets for winter babies
- Disposable diapers (100 or so per week)
- Cloth diapers. (If you go this route, you'll need upward of 24 diapers per day, though a stash of 48 will make your life easier. Or if you're using a local diaper service, they will let you know how many you will need.)
- 2–4 boxes of baby wipes
- Twins' diaper bag
- 10–14 one-piece undershirts
- 10–14 one-piece pajamas and/or gowns
- 4–8 pairs of sock

- 4–6 hats
- 4–6 blanket sleepers for winter babies
- Baby wash and lotion (such as Earth Mama Angel Baby or Weleda)
- 1 portable tub. Think *assembly line* when bathing twins!
- 4–8 washcloths and towels
- Diaper rash ointment or coconut oil
- 2 thermometers
- 2 bulb syringes (such as NoseFrida)
- 6–14 bottles and nipples if you plan on bottle feeding
- 2–4 large cans of formula. You'll use approximately a can a week, but it's nice to have extra on hand.
- 1 bottle brush
- 6–12 burp cloths
- 4–8 bibs
- Twins' nursing pillow. It's great for breastfeeding *and* bottle feeding.
- 1 or 2 baby swings and/or bouncer chairs. It's very important to have safe places to put a baby down.
- 1 or 2 changing stations
- A nursing chair wide enough to handle tandem nursing if you are planning on breastfeeding

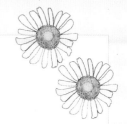

MY THIRD BIRTH

Luke Steven and Rocco Leroy
July 2, 2011
Twin Home Birth

I began working as a birth doula once my first set of twins, Birdie and Hazel, turned six months old. I was around pregnant women and birth constantly, but I thought I was done having my own babies. I adored them, but they were hard work, and my husband was definitely finished with having more kids. I then caught the baby-having bug, bad. I asked my husband for just one more baby. I romanticized the idea of one baby. My husband was convinced we would have twins again. I said, "Lighting doesn't strike twice." Famous last words.

After my twin girls, anything seemed easy to me. My husband wouldn't budge, but I would periodically ask him, hoping he'd change his mind. He didn't, but the universe was on my side. We used the rhythm method as birth control because I don't do well with hormone-based birth control. It didn't prove very effective in this instance. I remember my excitement and feelings of guilt when I got a positive pregnancy test. I knew my husband wasn't going to have the same level of excitement that I had. We were tired and overwhelmed already. For his birthday, I gave him the positive pregnancy test wrapped in a box. He was shocked and didn't really talk about it for a week or two. I guess he needed time to let the news sink in.

I was set on a home birth this time around and decided to once again get checked by my obstetrician before finding a home-birth midwife. I started to google "twins twice." What where my chances? One in three thousand, apparently. I lurked in a few online forums for parents-to-be expecting multiples. I guess I had a sixth sense that it might be twins again. My husband was already 100 percent convinced that we were having twins again. He came with me to the appointment. As soon as my obstetrician started the ultrasound, he knew what he was looking at. *Twins!* We laughed, we cried, and then we were silent. What the hell were we going to do? How would we break the news to my stepdaughter, Bella? I knew she loved her sisters but wasn't thrilled with the whole baby thing. Especially twins. Again.

This was the biggest shock of my entire life. It's hard to even describe the feeling. Everyone got used to the idea eventually. Most people didn't believe me at first. I remember being nervous right before my 18-week anatomy scan thinking that something was wrong with the babies. I over-researched things like vanishing twin syndrome, and it made my anxiety go through the roof. But while I was riding the train to the hospital for the scan, a set of teenage twin boys with the exact same voice sat across from me. I had an intense sense of relief wash over me. I knew at that moment, even before the ultrasound, that my babies were going to be okay, and that they were boys. I was right, and my husband was finally thrilled. He was going to have a son after four daughters. Two of them!

I decided to seek dual care for the duration of my pregnancy. I felt like I was cheating on my obstetrician, because I never told her my plan for a home birth. My midwife was only willing to deliver my twins at home if they were born after thirty-six weeks. I agreed that this was a good goal to reach in order to proceed with a safe home delivery. She was also thrilled that they were di/di (dizygotic, or fraternal, meaning they developed from two separate eggs that were fertilized by two separate sperm), which decreases some of the risks associated with a twin delivery. I reached the thirty-six-week goal and then some. I carried my boys to thirty-nine weeks and three days. I was walking around 5 cm dilated for weeks!

My obstetrician offered many times to break my water and get the show on the road. I was tempted. But I dreaded delivering in the hospital if it wasn't medically necessary. I cried every day for the last few weeks. It was hard carrying those boys so long, but it was worth it. I went into labor around 7 a.m. on July 2. I woke up and started contracting right away. My mother, aunt, and sister had all spent the night. My sister was in town to visit the new babies that I hadn't given birth to yet because no one thought I would carry them to forty weeks! It worked out perfectly that they were all there. They made the kids some breakfast and took them to the park while my husband called the midwife. My contractions were hard and fast. I knew that this was going to be a quick labor.

I hopped in the shower and let the hot water hit my back. The contractions came with lots of pressure. This labor felt different from my two previous labors. I felt in control and relaxed. I could manage the contractions, and I wasn't running from the pain. I was embracing them and actually enjoying it. I finally learned to trust my body and the process of giving birth. I had also supported quite a few births as a birth doula and witnessed the power and strength of our birthing bodies. I got out of the tub rather quickly, and it seemed like my midwife just magically appeared. I labored in my room for a bit and my midwife checked me. I was fully dilated. She asked me to stand because my bag of waters was bulging. I stood up, and with the next contraction my water broke. It was a huge relief. I decided to lay on the bed to rest between contractions. Then I felt like trying to push a little. I was laughing and joking between contractions. I pushed Luke out at 10:05 a.m., just three short hours after labor began. I remember pushing him out and thinking what a huge relief it was. I then quickly remembered that I had to push out another baby too. My contractions slowed down a bit, and it took a little longer to get Rocco out. He was born in the caul (the amniotic sac) at 10:51 a.m., forty-six minutes later.

I remember saying how easy the birth was right after giving birth. I really enjoyed these births. I was so happy that I was able to give birth to my sons at home and that they were huge and healthy. Luke was 8 pounds (3.6 kg) and Rocco was 7 pounds, 9 ounces (3.4 kg). They nursed like champs. Soon after I gave birth, my girls came back from the park and climbed into bed with me to meet their new brothers. It was so sweet that it brings tears to my eyes just thinking about it. I had the perfect birth. I deserved at least one orgasmic birth, right? Hah! I am so grateful to my amazing midwife, who agreed to stand by my side. I really did not have many people supporting my decision to have a home birth with twins. She will always hold a special place in my heart. I am so glad I could experience the beauty of a calm and peaceful birth.

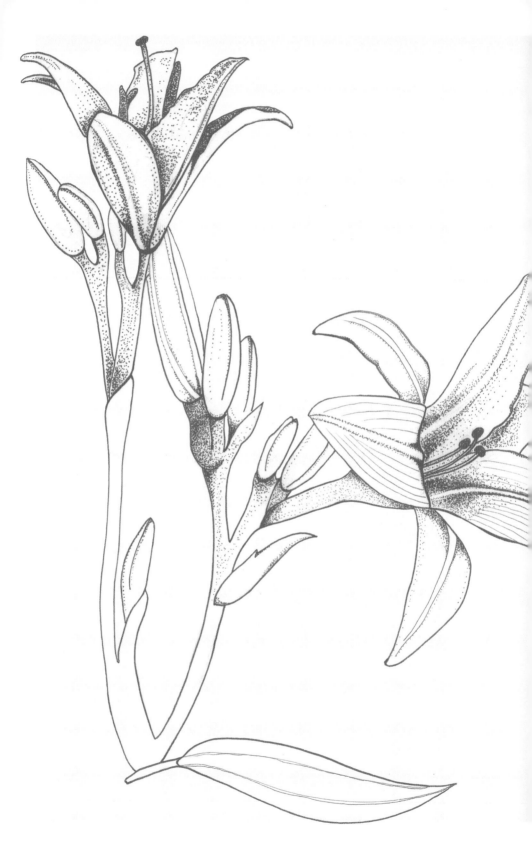

Part Three

The Fourth Trimester and Beyond

Fourth Trimester Healing

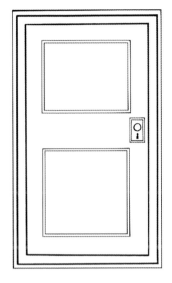
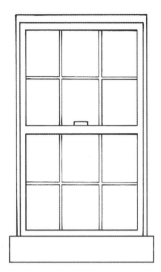

YOUR MAGNIFICENT BODY IS GOING TO BIRTH A HUMAN being. It deserves rest and care after accomplishing this astounding feat. You may end up having a vaginal birth or a cesarean birth. Both are considered giving *birth*, by the way. Some babies come out the door, and others come out the window. Everyone's body heals differently. Recovery is typically easier and quicker if you have a vaginal delivery, but not always. One of my birth doula clients has had two babies with me, one born vaginally and the other through cesarean birth. She found that her cesarean birth was an easier recovery process. Remember, everyone's childbirth and postpartum experience is unique, like a snowflake.

When I gave birth to my first baby, I felt wildly unprepared for the postpartum journey. Many things happened to me that no one had told me about or cared to share with me. I found out the hard way. I wish that I had gone into my postpartum journey better prepared and less in denial. We prepare so much for the childbirth part that we often forget there's going to be a fourth trimester. The fourth trimester is the time during which your body is recovering from childbirth while you are learning to become a parent. It's major!

Here are some of the things that I wish someone had told me.

Your empty tummy feels like a gelatinous mound of flesh. It is an odd and unexpected feeling. Your organs feel like they are shifting about. Your core feels almost nonexistent. You may find some comfort in a postpartum compression band. I tied a scarf around my postpartum tummy for just a touch of added support. It can help take the pressure off your lower back. Be extra gentle with your tummy if you are recovering from a cesarean birth. Most of the stitches from your incision will dissolve nowadays, but some obstetricians may use staples, and you will need to have them removed.

You bleed. I remember after my first birth, the midwife told me that I should make sure I don't have any blood clots larger than the size of my fist. My *fist?!* Really? Every time I stood up during those first few days, I'd feel a warm gush of blood. Postpartum bleeding (lochia) is heaviest up until ten days postpartum. You will have lochia up to four to six weeks postpartum. You also bleed vaginally if you have a cesarean birth. Those ugly mesh undies you get from the hospital are phenomenal. They hold a big old sanitary napkin nicely. I don't know anyone who doesn't like them. Don't worry, home birthers, you can also order some with your home birth kit. Another option is wearing adult diapers. I'm not kidding. Birth is juicy, people.

You'll probably be very hungry. I was starving 24/7. I remember the first meal after I gave birth more vividly than I remember the actual birth.

EXPERT TIP

on Postpartum Bleeding

by Carrie Perry, *postpartum doula and mother*

Lochia should get lighter and lighter as days and weeks pass postpartum. If there is a day when bleeding becomes heavier, it is a sign that you've done too much!

Lochia

Originating from a Greek word meaning "relating to childbirth," lochia is vaginal discharge during the postpartum period that consists of blood and tissue from the uterine lining.

It was lasagna, in case you were wondering. I ate a portion big enough to feed five grown men. If people want to visit you postpartum, make sure they come with food. A meal train is a wonderful way for your friends and family to support you.

If you are recovering from a cesarean birth, you will not be able to eat until six to eight hours post-delivery. You may not even be hungry right away, because you will likely be nauseous and gassy for up to forty-eight hours. When all of this subsides, you will become ravenous. Consider eating anti-inflammatory foods such as leafy greens, nuts, and berries.

You may have stitches in your vagina. Most first-time vaginal birthers will have some perineal tearing. If you do, it will sting every time you pee during those first few days postpartum. A mixture of witch hazel and warm water in a peri bottle will become your best friend. Squirt your vagina while peeing and you will get sweet relief and no stinging.

If you had a surgical delivery, you may have a very sore and painful incision site. Please take your painkillers. You just had major abdominal surgery. A big mistake that people make is skipping the pain meds and becoming filled with overwhelming pain and anxiety. Be aware that the pain can actually prevent your breast milk from coming in if you are hoping to breastfeed. Please ask for assistance in finding positions that do not put pressure on your incision. Typically, a side-lying position feels the most comfortable post-surgery.

The dreaded postpartum poop is no joke. When I had just pushed a baby out of my body, the idea of pushing anything else out made me think I could physically come undone. I didn't want to bust a stitch.

Snack

Set up a snack area in all your nursing/infant-feeding locations. Make sure it's within an arm's length away so you can easily grab it with a baby or babies in your arms. Think raw almonds, dried fruit, or avocado toast. Hydration is also of utmost importance. Always have a full glass of water nearby.

Chestfeeding

Chestfeeding is a gender-neutral term used by some trans men and gender-nonconforming individuals for nursing their babies.

Hydrate to avoid constipation. Take a stool softener if necessary. If you have a C-birth, they will send you home with stool softeners to combat the constipation from the pain medication.

Your breasts/chest may go through a massive transformation around two to five days after birth. My partner left briefly to go to the store and returned to find a pair of hot (literally) gigantic torpedo breasts. They were so engorged and painful that it took me by surprise. Why do people just refer to this process as when "your milk comes in"? That phrase seems so benign in contrast to what actually happens to your body. The discomfort should only be temporary and normally subsides within twenty-four hours. This may not happen so drastically to you, but if it does, aren't you glad that you aren't alone for the ride?

If you are planning on breastfeeding or chestfeeding your baby/babies, there are a few things to know immediately postpartum to help aid in breastfeeding success. Try to nurse your baby within the first hour after delivery. Babies usually tank out for a long stretch after being alive for a few hours. You will be producing colostrum, also known as *liquid gold* (see page 160). Newborns only need the littlest bit of colostrum

on Healing the Perineum

by Robin Rose Bennett, *writer, green witch, herbalist, wisewoman, and founder of Wisewoman Healing Ways*

This depends on the woman and what she is feeling, of course. A good general nourishing infusion such as linden blossoms, alternating with red clover blossom infusions, can be helpful in providing an abundant supply of nervous system–soothing and –strengthening minerals, anti-inflammatory compounds, and circulation-enhancing bioflavonoids. Lady's mantle (*Alchemilla vulgaris*) tincture, about 20–35 drops in water or tea, is a generous ally in helping a woman get a sense of physical and emotional balance back after birth (or any major hormonal experience).

A great sitz bath recipe to heal the perineum can be made with ½ cup each of any of the following herbs: comfrey leaf (15 g), calendula flowers (113 g), witch hazel leaves (12 g) or bark (38 g), yarrow flowers (15 g), and/or plantain leaves (18 g). Place herbs in a ½-gallon (2 L) jar and pour boiling water over them.

because their stomach is only the size of a marble. That first feed helps to get their bowels to pass that thick, tar-like meconium (see page 177).

Spend lots of time skin to skin with your baby. Feed your newborn in a semi-reclined or laid-back position. Nursing may be uncomfortable at first. This is probably the first time in your life that your nipples have had this much action. Even if the baby's latch is perfect, your nipples may still be tender. However, shooting pain and bloody nipples are not normal, and you should seek out the support of a lactation specialist. If something doesn't feel right, please ask for help. You are learning right along with your baby. I breastfed six children, and each child's breastfeeding journey was different. They had very different issues and struggles. I had one client struggle a great deal with breastfeeding her firstborn child. Her next birth was twins, and the breastfeeding experience was "easy"

Cracked Nipples

For healing cracked nipples, I recommend using a homemade saline rinse (½ teaspoon [2.5 g] sea salt in 8 ounces [235 ml] warm water). After each feed, rinse your nipples fully with the saline rinse and let them air-dry. If your baby doesn't like the salty taste, rinse with warm water before the next feed. This remedy really works at accelerating the healing process.

in comparison. You can never anticipate exactly how it will unfold. (For more information on feeding, see page 159.)

The postpartum body can be a challenge for some. You may not slip into your pre-pregnancy jeans right away, or perhaps ever again. That's okay. Your body spent all that time growing and nurturing your baby; it also deserves the time to recover. Invest in some stretchy and comfy clothing. This is not the time to start a restrictive fad diet. There is no race to lose the baby weight. Why would you want to do that to yourself? Eat healthy and nourishing foods to allow your body to heal. I detest the companies that prey on our postpartum bodies, trying to shrink and wrap them into unrealistic shapes. A body that is dimpled in cellulite and stretch marks is the canvas that brought forth new life. Your body deserves to be worshiped and honored.

PELVIC FLOOR HEALTH AND HEALING

Pelvic floor health after you have a baby is extremely important. My daughter is well over a year old, and I still squirt when I sneeze. I can't jump without wetting my pants. I had to take CrossFit off my list of post-partum exercise picks. This is one of those things that rarely gets talked about before you have a baby. You do all the prep work to have a healthy pregnancy and childbirth, but what do you do to take care of your body after it's done all the work? My biggest fear is that after birthing six babies, my uterus is going to fall out. Literally.

Kegel Exercises

We always hear about doing your Kegel exercises during pregnancy. Well, I'm a big advocate for doing Kegels *after* childbirth too. A Kegel is a contract-and-release exercise to strengthen the pelvic floor, which childbirth can weaken. A weakened pelvic floor can lead to incontinence; a prolapsed uterus, bladder, or anus; and/or decreased sensation. You may wonder how to find your pelvic floor muscles to do a Kegel; put your focus on the sensation of holding back your pee or holding in a fart. During those first couple of weeks postpartum, I encourage you to do fifty Kegel exercises every time you feed your baby. *Hold. Release. Hold. Release.* Play around with the speed of the Kegels. I named the fast Kegels *lightning Kegels* and the slow ones *turtle Kegels.* There are many pelvic floor exercise devices on the market today. Do some research and speak to your care provider. I strongly encourage you to seek out the services of a pelvic physical therapist if you are experiencing incontinence or loss of sensation.

Yoni Eggs

I am a beginning yoni egg user. I recently gave birth to my sixth baby, and I know that my pelvic floor needs love and attention. You may be wondering why I would even consider shoving a jade egg on a string up my vagina? Well to start, yoni eggs are popular in my local natural healing and yoga community. Curiosity got the best of me, because I have heard only positive experiences from friends and colleagues. Yoni eggs have been used for more than five thousand years to access sexual power and health. The idea of focusing energy on my vagina was powerful because I would be honoring a part of my body that was used to bring life into the world. Doing Kegel exercises with your jade yoni egg will strengthen the

BREASTFEEDING ESSENTIALS

by LaShanda Dandrich, *IBCLC, postpartum doula, and mother*

Your mammary glands! After all, we are mammals and meant to feed our young through our marvelous mammary organs. I know that doesn't sound glamourous, but it is nature at its finest.

Breastfeeding (or breastmilk) works by the way our hormones function in our body. When the baby leaves our body, also known as *birth*, followed by the placenta leaving the body, a hormone shift happens that starts continued lactation. The milk produced is meant to feed the human(s) we have created who are now on the outside of the body.

I emphasize this to say that if you are aware (sometimes we are unaware) of any hormonal issues you have had during or prior to your pregnancy, you will want to speak with an IBCLC (International Board Certified Lactation Consultant) when thinking about breastfeeding your baby. This includes any surgeries to the breast or nipples and any developmental abnormalities of the breast.

Even if you don't have these issues, I highly recommend taking a prenatal breastfeeding class and learning about the physiological process of making and keeping a good milk supply. Breastfeeding may not look like it does in the books or what it looks like for your sister, friend, cousin, or neighbor. Breastfeeding is a relationship between you and your child(ren).

One of the other important components to the breastfeeding equation is, of course, your baby (babies).

Though breastfeeding is a natural process, keep in mind it is a "new" way for your infant to eat. And they, just like you, have to learn this new process. So even though infants come out of the womb expecting to latch onto a breast, they do not know what type of breast and nipple they are going to encounter. It is very helpful to learn the proper way to latch your baby, how it should feel (painless), and ways to help your little human achieve that.

Since this is new for your infant, allow for a grace period. Give your infant time to learn to "trust" the breast. Take into consideration things they are adjusting to:

- Latching wider onto a breast (they have been practicing on a tiny hand)

- Learning to suck, swallow, and breathe at the breast

- How long to feed until they feel satiated

- How long a feed is and how many times to eat in the twenty-four-hour day

- Adjusting to life outside of the womb

Again, I highly encourage taking a breastfeeding class so you will know the answers, and what is "normal" for the average healthy full-term infant.

If you have a premature infant, or if at any time you feel that breast-feeding is not working well, please reach out to your pediatrician *and* a lactation consultant to help you *both* figure out what works.

You may not have been expecting to see support under "Essentials," but it is really my number one recommendation to all breastfeeding families for getting breastfeeding off to a good start. Preparation for breast-feeding and building your support team has to start in pregnancy. Make sure your health care professional(s) and birth team are on board with supporting breastfeeding. Have the discussion about what your preferences are in labor (drug interventions, natural process of birth) and also what is expected right after birth. Review hospital protocols if you are birthing in a hospital. Skin to skin should be practiced as soon as possible to help the infant tune into the natural instincts to look for the breast.

Beyond that is the immediate support. Your partner should attend the breastfeeding class as well. It sometimes takes a team to feed a baby in the beginning, and having everyone aware of the process is very helpful. Grandparents can also attend, or you can consider purchasing a book for them to read. Many of our parents come from a generation when breast-feeding was not encouraged, and because of that, they sometimes do not trust that the infant will be properly fed. This can also be true of partners, and in both situations, it can put a lot of stress on the lactating parent.

Do not assume that the OB, pediatrician, doula, or night nurse are breastfeeding friendly either. Breastfeeding friendly does not only consist of a kind "hang in there" attitude coupled with a "you can always give formula" comment. Support means being able to assess the situation and recommend the appropriate course of action to help achieve your original goal. Many times breastfeeding does not succeed due to lack of confidence and support, not from not having enough supply.

The profession of lactation consultant is fairly new, and we need many more to support breastfeeding dyads. In addition to finding an IBCLC (which can be done via ILCA.org), you can create a support network for yourself. I like to say if you are training for a marathon, you don't hang out with couch potatoes. If your goal is to breastfeed your infant, find those who fully support your goal.

Reach out to your local WIC (Women, Infants, and Children) office or La Leche League group. If you are not sure where to start, Facebook has many local breastfeeding support groups where you can ask questions of peers.

Pelvic Floor

The pelvic floor is the group of muscles that act as a supportive sling in the lower pelvis. The muscles surround the vaginal opening, the anus, and the urethra. These muscles keep your uterus inside your body and help you control your urine and bowel movements.

pelvic floor and increase sensitivity. Jade is less porous than other stones, which is why it is the top yoni egg choice. Jade is the stone of health and abundance, known for revitalizing healing. Please consult with your care provider if you are unsure of the safety of this practice.

POSTPARTUM EMOTIONS

I mentioned a lot of the physical changes that may happen immediately postpartum, but what about the emotional transformation that you may undergo? No one prepared me for the crushing responsibility of becoming someone's parent. We hear the term *baby blues* thrown around very loosely. A few of my friends shared that they were a little weepy postpartum, but they never really divulged the *real* emotional processing that they actually went through. It's almost as if they felt shame or embarrassment and didn't want to share it out loud. Nothing will rock your world more than having a baby. *Nothing.* Mood swings, crying fits, insomnia, irritability, regret, joy, shame, guilt, inadequacy, and sadness are all normal postpartum responses. This emotional roller coaster usually comes to an end around two to three weeks postpartum. If it doesn't, this would be a good time to reach out for some additional support. There is no shame in asking for help. I had my therapist on speed dial after I gave birth to my first set of twins. If you are feeling suicidal and unable to care for yourself or your newborn, reach out for help immediately.

POSTPARTUM SELF-CARE

When I visit doula clients for their postpartum visit, I walk into all sorts of scenarios. The one thing that I encounter over and over again is new parents doing way too much. At a recent postpartum visit, a client was on her hands and knees scrubbing the kitchen floor less than a week postpartum. I gently grabbed her by the hand and walked her to the bedroom. She nursed the baby in bed while I massaged her feet and then brought her a cup of tea. I told her that she deserves this time to heal. She is worthy of self-care. And who really cares if the kitchen floor is dirty? Be easy on yourself postpartum. Call on your village to support and nourish you after your little one arrives. Most friends and family want to help. Take advantage of their offering of support when the luster of a new baby is shining bright.

POSTPARTUM PREFERENCES

Everyone focuses so much on the birth part that planning for the postpartum period often gets neglected. It is well worth your time and energy to create postpartum preferences. What are you hoping your postpartum period will look like? Set clear boundaries and discuss your wishes before your little one arrives.

In the hospital or birthing center:
○ Are you choosing to delay newborn care procedures for one hour to help facilitate bonding?
○ What are your plans for infant feeding?
○ Is there lactation support available?
○ Will the baby be rooming in with you?

POSTPARTUM HERBAL BATH

My home birth midwife gave me clearance almost immediately postpartum for an herbal bath. Sorry, C-birthers, if you've had a surgical delivery you will have to wait a bit longer for your obstetrician to give you the go-ahead. Herbal baths are great for healing sore vaginas, hemorrhoids, and tearing. The herbs I selected are also helpful in aiding the healing of your baby's umbilical stump. My baby and I took our ceremonial first herbal bath together.

Purchase a drawstring muslin bag to put your herbs in. Hang the herbal blend over your faucet so the warm water runs through into your bathtub. Once the tub is full, toss in the closed bag filled with herbs.

Add ½ cup (130 g) Himalayan sea salt directly to the bathtub while filling with warm water. Fill the bag with:

¼ cup (8 g) dried comfrey leaves
¼ cup (7 g) lavender
¼ cup (14 g) dried red raspberry leaves
¼ cup (14 g) dried yarrow flowers

Enjoy.

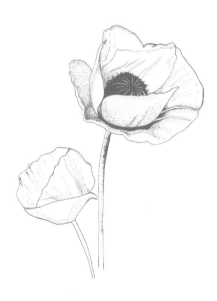

Support at home:

○ Who is your support team (family, friends, a postpartum doula, etc.)?

○ What are your plans for nourishment?

○ Consider having visiting hours so you don't overwhelm yourself and/or the new baby. Keep visits short and sweet. No one should come over empty-handed, either.

○ Who will help with the household chores?

POSTPARTUM NUTRITION

Eat hearty, simple foods. Staying nourished so your body can heal is essential for getting those hormones back in check. Here are some simple suggestions for food to indulge in and foods to avoid. Remember, if you are breastfeeding, you will need to consume 300 to 500 extra calories a day to sustain the needs of your new baby. Avoid empty calories.

Nourishing foods:

Almond butter. High in protein and awesome for making energy balls or adding to a smoothie.

Almonds. Great for snacking and keeping on your bedside table. High in protein.

Avocados. Full of good fat and a great snack for energy postpartum.

Berries. Full of antioxidants. Eat them by the handful or add them to a smoothie.

Bone broth. Jam-packed with nutrients and perfect for healing. Preparing and storing some in your freezer will serve you well. See page 155.

Probiotics

Consider taking a probiotic supplement post-delivery. You will be given antibiotics during your surgery that can wipe out healthy gut flora. Help along your recovery by boosting your immune system. Be sure to run this by your care provider.

Homemade chicken and root vegetable soup. There is a reason that Gramma's homemade chicken soup always made you feel better. Collagen is wonderful for healing after both vaginal and surgical deliveries. Throw in some root vegetables, which are full of beta-carotene.

Fish. Wild salmon and sardines are high in omega-3 fatty acids, which are important to include in a healthy postpartum diet. Omega-3 fatty acids have been found to lower overall rates of postpartum depression.

Flaxseed oil. High in omega-3 fatty acids.

Green smoothies. See page 33.

Leafy greens. Filled with vitamin A, which is good for you and baby. Greens have antioxidants that are good for your heart. Leafy greens are also excellent blood builders, which are extremely important if you experienced blood loss during childbirth. Stock up on spinach, kale, and mustard greens.

Nettle infusion. Steeping dried nettles in hot water for eight hours makes a blood-building tonic that does wonders for your energy. Nettles can enrich and increase breastmilk production. See page 156.

Vegan Lentil Soup. See page 154.

VEGAN LENTIL SOUP

by Carrie Perry, *postpartum doula and mother*

I use 4 cubes Rapunzel brand "herbs and sea salt" boullon with 8 cups (1.9 L) water. No additional salt. Also, the thyme I use is from a friend's garden in Guyana. It's so special and gives my soup a unique flavor. *Makes 6 to 8 servings.*

2 cups (384 g) green lentils, rinsed
8 cups (1.9 L) vegetable broth
3 carrots, chopped
1 small to medium-size onion, chopped
4 cloves garlic, minced
1 tablespoon (3 g) French thyme
1 bunch spinach
1–2 teaspoons (5–10 ml) balsamic vinegar
Salt to taste

Combine lentils, broth, carrots, onion, garlic, and thyme in a heavy-bottomed pot. Bring to a boil over high heat. Reduce heat to low and cover with a tight-fitting lid. Simmer, covered, for 2 hours. Alternatively, use a slow cooker on low for 8 hours.

Add spinach and balsamic vinegar. Cook an additional 10 minutes. Salt to taste. Serve warm.

BONE BROTH
IN A SLOW COOKER

You can help aid your postpartum healing process with this easy recipe for bone broth. I recommend using organic, hormone-free, free-range chicken. *Makes 4 to 6 servings.*

1 organic roasted chicken carcass
1 tablespoon (15 g) Himalayan sea salt
1 medium onion, halved
4 cloves garlic, smashed
1 large organic carrot, chopped
2 stalks celery with leaves, chopped
2 bay leaves
2 tablespoons (30 ml) Bragg apple cider vinegar
8 cups (1.9 L) filtered water

Combine ingredients in a slow cooker and cook, covered, on low for 24 hours.

Let cool and pour through a strainer. Drink immediately or store in glass mason jars in the refrigerator for a few days or the freezer for up to a year.

MAKING A NETTLE TONIC

by Carriage House Birth, *Childbirth Educators and Doulas*

Carriage House Birth makes this simple infusion. It's quick to make, keeps for a few days, and is effortless to use. It's great for your kids to sip on too. Nettles for health, nettles for our souls, nettles for life! *Makes about 1 quart (945 ml).*

1   Bring 1 quart (1 L) water to a boil and let cool slightly.
2   Add 1 cup (90 g) dried nettles to a thick glass quart-size (1 L) jar (make sure the glass will take the heat and not break).
3   Pour water into the jar and put the lid on tightly.
4   Leave to infuse for 5–10 hours or even overnight; the infusion should be as dark as Coca-Cola.
5   Strain out the leaves.

You now have a super-rich and beneficial elixir you can drink throughout the day. Aim for at least 2–3 cups (470–705 ml) if not all of the drink. The nettle infusion does not have a long shelf life and may start to spoil after 36 hours, depending on room temperature. We keep our infusions in the fridge, where they can last for 3 days. If you have any left after that, pour on your hair in the shower and let it sit for a few minutes, then rinse for an herbal hair-healing treatment.

Drink chilled or on ice! It tastes awful warm. It can also be mixed with a stone fruit juice such as peach or mango.

Foods to avoid postpartum:

Sugar. Stay away from empty calories and refined sugar. Sugar is the devil. Stick to natural sugar by eating fruits instead.

Booze. You may have been waiting nine months to start drinking alcohol again, but it really has no benefits to you or your baby. Stick to an occasional glass of red wine if you must. No need to pump and dump if you are only having a glass. Moderate drinking and breastfeeding don't mix well. Try having a hangover with a newborn—it might be the last drink you take!

Caffeine. It's sometimes hard to practice what you preach. I limited my coffee intake to 1 cup (235 ml) a day. Too much caffeine can trigger anxiety in you and cause restlessness in a breastfed baby.

Dairy. Dairy is the most common allergy culprit for newborns. If you're breastfeeding, consider limiting your dairy intake.

Spicy foods. Breastfed babies may object to spicy foods.

Wheat. Wheat is full of sugar, and it can cause blood sugar to spike rapidly. Wheat also contains gluten, which is hard for most people to digest. Gluten sensitivity can cause adverse effects in many people.

Beef. Red meat is high in saturated fat, which raises blood cholesterol. Meat today is pumped full of hormones and antibiotics. I personally avoid *all* red meat.

Raw garlic and onions. They may cause gas for your newborn if you're breastfeeding.

Breastfeeding/ Infant Feeding

BREASTS AND BOTTLES ARE BOTH FEEDING VESSELS. BOTH feed your baby. You will end up using one or the other, or maybe both. My goal is not to pressure you into breastfeeding or to make you feel bad if you cannot or decide not to breastfeed. Human milk is best for human babies, but it is not always possible. My goal in this section is to offer you information to help you prepare to potentially breastfeed/chestfeed.

Consider meeting with a lactation consultant or attending a La Leche League meeting before you actually give birth. Take a look at your nipple anatomy to see if you have flat or inverted nipples. You may be able to ask questions now and prepare before your little one arrives.

If you are planning on breastfeeding, let your support team know and include your wishes on your birth preferences sheet. If you are delivering in a hospital, it is also important to let the staff know you are breastfeeding. Any necessary supplemental feeding can be administered via oral syringe. You don't want to confuse your little one right out of the gate. Please have your care provider or a lactation specialist observe your newborn's latch before you leave your place of delivery.

You can stock up on a few things to prepare for breastfeeding:

- 2 or more comfortable nursing bras
- Easy-access clothing/robe
- Breast pump
- Rocking chair/glider
- Nipple balm
- Nursing pillow. This is optional; sometimes it's essential and sometimes it's irrelevant. I absolutely needed one with my premature twins, but didn't use one with my last baby.

In those first few weeks postpartum, please don't invite anyone who will be uncomfortable seeing your breasts over to your home. You don't have time for that. Your focus will be on being topless and skin to skin with your new baby.

LET YOUR NEWBORN SET THE SCHEDULE

You can't nurse too often during those first two weeks. Aim to nurse ten to twelve times a day. Some babies nurse every hour. Wait for your baby to show signs of hunger. These signs include lip smacking, rooting (a reflex that happens when the corner of a newborn's mouth is touched and she turns her head toward that touch, opens her mouth, and begins to make sucking motions), or hands/fists in mouth. If your baby is super sleepy, you can try expressing colostrum and rubbing your nipple by his cheek. I rubbed a cool washcloth on the hands and feet to wake up one of my babies. I know that sounds cruel, but I had a very sleepy newborn who was slow to gain weight and needed the extra feeding. I had clients tell me that they had to change their baby's diaper before each feeding in order to wake her up fully. The old diaper-changing trick works for many sleepy newborns. Try feeding your newborn at least every two hours during the day and then every four hours at night.

One of the biggest concerns for most new breastfeeding parents is wondering if your baby is getting enough to eat. You don't get to see the amount and measure it in a bottle when you are breastfeeding. This can be problematic for some people. Make sure you can see your baby swallowing while feeding. Check for wet diapers. Those first few days,

Colostrum

Colostrum is the antibody-rich first milk that your body produces to help protect your newborn baby from disease. You will produce colostrum for an average of two to five days before you start producing mature breastmilk. This liquid gold is creamy or yellowish in color and thicker than mature milk. It is low in fat and high in carbohydrates and protein. Colostrum acts as a laxative to help your newborn baby start moving her bowels. Its main purpose is to boost the immune system and prevent disease. Mature milk is higher in volume and aids digestion, develops the brain, and gives your baby energy.

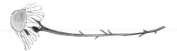

on Breastfeeding

by Robin Rose Bennett, *writer, green witch, herbalist, wisewoman, and founder of Wisewoman Healing Ways*

Fennel seed tea works well for many women, is tasty, and relieves gas, too. Bitter-tasting hops tea or tincture is a traditional remedy to bring down a plentiful supply of breast milk. Regular use during pregnancy of red raspberry leaf and nettle leaf infusions also helps ensure plentiful breast milk later, as well as helping with a healthy pregnancy and delivery.

you will only have one or two. When your milk comes in around after two to five days, it should be around five or six diapers a day. You will also be bringing your baby to the pediatrician for a weight check to make sure he is gaining weight properly. Many babies will lose a small percentage of their birth weight initially, so don't be alarmed. If you are concerned about anything, please reach out for advice and support.

FAVORITE POSITIONS FOR BREASTFEEDING

Laid-Back Breastfeeding: Lie down in a semi-reclining position. Now lay your baby down tummy to tummy. Let your baby find his own way to your nipple.

Cradle Hold: This is the classic breastfeeding hold, in which your baby's head rests in the crook of your arm on the side that you will be breast-feeding from. Your other hand will be free if you need to be hands-on with latching your baby on. "Nipple to nose" is an extremely helpful reminder in those early latching days.

Football Hold: This was the only position that I could breastfeed my 35-weeker newborn twins in. It enabled them to open their mouths wider for a much more efficient latch. I also recommend this position for post-cesarean delivery because the baby stays off your incision site. Tuck your baby's legs and feet underneath your arm, on the same side you are nursing from. Imagine a football player tucking a football (hence the name).

Side-Lying Position: Lie down on your side facing parallel to your baby. Pull your baby in. Latch on and snuggle. This position saved my life during those sleep-deprived newborn days. I loved not having to physically get up out of bed in the middle of the night. I'd just pull my baby over and feed. This is also a great position post-cesarean because it stays off the incision.

NIPPLES

Sore nipples are pretty common in the beginning of your breastfeeding experience. Some experts say that it shouldn't hurt at all. I call bullshit on that. It's probably the first time in your life that your nipples have had that most action. If they start cracking and bleeding, please reach out to have a lactation counselor or an International Board Certified Lactation Consultant (IBCLC) assess the latch. Sometimes it can be as simple asreadjusting the latch, or perhaps it is something more complicated like a tongue tie.

Tongue Tie

A tongue tie is a short frenulum (in this case, the piece of skin connecting the tongue to the bottom of the mouth or gums) that restricts tongue mobility. Sometimes a tongue tie can affect latching and/or milk intake.

MASTITIS

Please keep a lookout for some of the flu-like symptoms of mastitis, which is an infection of the breast tissue. It's most common during the first few months after birth, but it can happen up to two years after birth. It happened to me *twice* when my youngest daughter was thirteen months old. And I thought I was out of the woods! Mastitis is no joke. I wasn't even planning on mentioning it in this book until my good boob turned bad. I have never in my life been taken out in such a quick and vicious fashion. It all started with a literal pain in the boob. It felt like I had been dropkicked suddenly. I spiked a fever, got the full body shakes, and developed a screaming headache. There was pus coming out of my boob. I know, gross! I spent the next forty-eight hours in bed wondering if my husband should transfer me to the hospital. I used lots of natural healing remedies and antibiotics prescribed by my doctor, and twenty-four hours later I was recovering.

BREAST PUMPS

There are many ways to feed your new baby. Some parents choose to exclusively pump and feed their baby breastmilk in bottles. You are going to do whatever works for you and your family. During the first few weeks postpartum, it may or may not be helpful to pump occasionally to relieve engorgement. You can store this milk. Please don't overdo it, though. Pumping too much too soon will make your body think that you have to produce much more milk than you actually need. This may cause issues such as plugged ducts, engorgement, or mastitis. Once your wee one is a bit older, you may want to add pumping into your daily routine because it can be helpful to have a little stash of milk if you are hoping to sneak away for a yoga class or a baby-free lunch with friends. It's your freedom! Sometimes it's nice to have your partner or a friend feed the baby while you nap. I waited until three to four weeks postpartum before I started

on Healing Mastitis

by Loveday Why, *writer, healer, coach, and founder of wild-and-good.com*

This turbocharged honey is essential for times when you are feeling under the weather or are fighting a low-level infection and would prefer not to use antibiotics. It uses the wonder root turmeric alongside ginger, honey, and coconut oil to offer anti-inflammatory, antibacterial, and antifungal support. You can take a teaspoon a day or spread it onto toast in the morning. If you are struggling with mastitis and are searching for remedies, this is partly what I used to recover, and it was a delicious medicine!

½ tablespoon (7 g) coconut oil
½ cup (120 ml) honey
½ tablespoon (4 g) finely grated turmeric
1 tablespoon (5 g) finely grated ginger

Melt coconut oil and honey together. Stir all the ingredients together and store in a covered glass jar at room temperature. You will find that the ginger and turmeric rise to the top, so simply stir before using.

pumping, and if you are hoping to exclusively breastfeed, I would recommend holding off for that amount of time.

Pumping in the beginning can be discouraging. You barely get any milk. Don't fret though—this is completely normal. When you first introduce pumping, you're sending the message to your body to start producing more milk. Picking the same time every day to pump will signal the body to start producing more and more milk. Pumping once a day is sufficient for building a little stash of breastmilk. If you are planning on going back to work, you will pump for every missed feeding.

The hardest part about pumping for me was relaxing. I hated having a machine with tubes and cords connected to my breasts. Practicing a few times a week or every day can be helpful because it will become less and less uncomfortable. I always have a bunch of photographs of my baby nursing on my phone to look at while pumping to help with my milk letdown. I call it looking at my nursing porn.

SUPPLEMENTING

Breastfeeding alone may not cut it. I needed to supplement with both my sets of twins. They were struggling to gain weight and needed a little help. There is no shame in supplementing. We are all doing the best we can. I was fortunate enough to be provided with donor breastmilk from one of my best friends, who had an extremely abundant supply. You can research human milk banks and/or milk sharing groups in your area. Formula is another option for supplementing. Please research the best type of formula for your baby.

BOTTLES

Don't buy a million bottles until you know which one your baby will like. I recommend buying three different brands and trying them all out. I call it bottle play. It took almost six bottles to find one my firstborn would take. She was also a boob addict and wasn't sold on being away from me for a second.

OWN IT

I want to be very clear that the suggestions that I have shared may not work for you or your family. Please don't give yourself guilt if things don't go as you had initially planned. You need to create your own feeding goals to fit your family's individual needs and own them. There is no right or wrong. Don't allow anyone to judge you for your choices. I know many extremely healthy formula-fed babies and many healthy exclusively breastfed babies. I know people who breastfed their baby for one week and people who breastfed their child for seven years.

MANAGING VISITORS

Setting boundaries and relaying your needs are essential for managing visitors postpartum. Choose your guest list carefully. Who is really there to help you? The last thing that you should be doing is playing host/hostess to friends and family on little to no sleep. You are healing and navigating infant feeding. My rule was that anyone who was uncomfortable seeing my bare breasts couldn't come over. I also believe that no one should ever come over empty-handed. Food and/or diapers are always welcome. Consider setting visiting hours. This ensures that no one overstays their welcome. Remind your guests to wash their hands upon entering your home and to avoid coming over if they are ill.

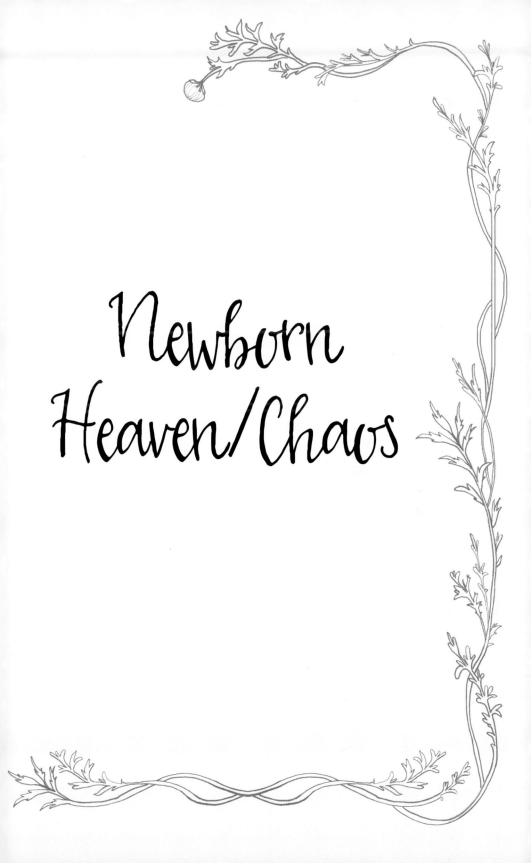

Newborn
Heaven/Chaos

WELCOMING A NEWBORN CAN CERTAINLY INCLUDE A roller coaster of emotions. Learning to surrender and embrace the chaos and unpredictability of those first few weeks and months will help you have a positive experience. Embrace chaos. Take deep cleansing breaths and nap when you can. This phase feels like it lasts an eternity when you're in it, but it goes by lightning fast.

SELF-CARE

Practicing self-care is challenging as a parent to a newborn. That little bundle of love can take up all your energy and attention. I remember finding it hard to even take a shower or go to the bathroom when I wanted to. I had to remind myself to eat, and I was lucky if my teeth were brushed that day.

Self-care is going to look different now that you are a parent. Self-care pre-baby may have meant going to get a massage or yoga classes five times a week. Or perhaps it was being able to meditate for an hour to start each morning. Accepting that self-care won't look the same will help you surrender to the new flow of things.

Creating a ritual of self-care is essential if you want to be an effective parent. If you have no self-care, everything will start to fall apart. That includes your relationship (if you're in one), your sanity, and your health. I made sure that I was implementing simple self-care rituals every single day. Before my husband left for work, I made sure that I got ten minutes to myself in the bathroom. I would take a hot shower with a couple of drops of lavender oil. I pretended like it was my own little ten-minute spa day. I did this even if I had a house full of screaming babies. I knew that my partner could handle them for such a small window of time. If I did something for myself to start the day, I rarely ended up feeling over-whelmed or resentful. I got in my me time.

The most common form of self-care among my clients is exercise. I am constantly running into former doula clients at SoulCycle and hot yoga class. Exercise and yoga classes are short enough that you can sneak away without too much guilt.

Here are some simple ways to implement your self-care:

- Nourish yourself. Eat real food. Skip the sugary treat and make yourself a green smoothie (see page 33).
- Accept help. Stop trying to do it all by yourself.
- Ask for help. Asking for help shows strength.
- Exercise, even if it's only once or twice a week.
- Sleep. Take catnaps when your baby naps.
- Connect with nature. Put your feet in the dirt and look up at the sky. Or, my favorite, lie on the grass and gaze up at the treetops.
- Get fresh air. Five deep belly breaths can change your energy instantly.
- Use aromatherapy. I throw a few drops of my favorite essential oil in the diffuser, and it's a treat for my senses.
- Learn to set boundaries. Say no! Don't take on too many responsibilities.
- Meditate. Five minutes in the morning before your little one stirs is completely manageable most days.
- Practice a hobby. Do something that you love. It's important to have heart work outside of parenting.
- Go on a date night, if you have a partner or are looking for one.

Setting the intention to practice self-care during pregnancy will get you in the habit and will follow you into parenthood. Modeling self-care for your children is extremely important. It shows that you value yourself and will teach your children to value themselves too.

Multip

Multip is short for *multipara*, or a person who has given birth two or more times.

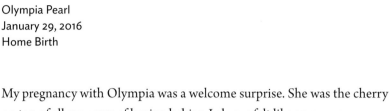

MY LAST BIRTH

Olympia Pearl
January 29, 2016
Home Birth

My pregnancy with Olympia was a welcome surprise. She was the cherry on top of all my years of having babies. I always felt like someone was missing from my beautiful madhouse. It was Olympia. I was very excited to welcome a singleton after birthing and juggling two sets of twins. My pregnancy was very challenging, and I am forever grateful to my partner and my doula partners (my doula wives!) for emotionally supporting me.

Being an experienced doula was both a blessing and a curse during this pregnancy. I had too many options and that felt very overwhelming at times. I was more anxious this pregnancy than I was with my first. I guess ignorance is bliss. But my anxiety seemed to melt away around thirty-five weeks, and I started to prepare and get excited to give birth to this baby. Olympia was very timely and labor really got going at forty weeks on the nose. I was having contractions on and off for a few days, but nothing too intense or worth really paying attention to. I went to bed and woke up around 2 a.m. having a few more contractions than usual. I timed a few and they seemed to be around seven to eight minutes apart. I texted my doula wives and told them that I was contracting but fine and trying to rest because I thought I was still really early. I texted my midwife at 2:25 a.m. just to give her a heads-up. I still hadn't even woken up my husband, Dan. A few minutes later I had a strong contraction and felt a sharp kick and popping sensation. My water broke. I woke up my husband. I called my midwife to let her know. Thank goodness she was already in transit to my house. She's pretty intuitive and sensed that things were moving fast and I was in denial.

At this point, things kicked into high gear. The contractions were definitely getting stronger. During one contraction, I was clutching a large chunk of rose quartz trying to breathe into it. The mantra "The power and intensity of your contractions cannot be stronger than you, because they are you" was running through my head. The next contraction was so strong that I threw the rock and thought, "F*$k this. *No.*" I kept thinking, "*How the hell can I get out of this?*" I had my husband pressing on my hips and sacrum but nothing was really helping. My midwife arrived and set up. The rest is a bit of a blur. I remember a few earth-shattering contractions and feeling like I was going to give birth to a Mack truck. My body spontaneously pushed twice, and Olympia shot out. I looked down and a baby slithered into my husband's waiting hands at 3:46 a.m. My doula wife/friend Samantha walked into my bedroom just in time to witness the birth of my placenta.

The birth was lightning fast and really intense. I swear my twin home birth was euphoric or even orgasmic compared to this. One of my big concerns about being a multip was having blood loss, but I ended up having very little bleeding and absolutely no tearing. The morning rolled around, and my kids slowly started to trickle into my bedroom. They were all wide-eyed and shocked that the baby had come while they were sleeping. It was sweet to see their excitement. My husband called our nanny/friend to come in case the kids woke up early. She helpfully kept them occupied for those first few hours after the birth. My other doula wife, Domino, came by with some delicious roasted chicken and cupcakes. She knows I have a sweet tooth. My friend Carrie, a postpartum doula, swung by with some lentil soup. She also came back the next week for a few hours here and there to help me juggle the baby. Our friend dropped off a lasagna that sustained me for days. My mother showed up in the early evening. And then my father and stepmother showed up and took the girls to dinner at the Museum of Modern Art and a sleepover at their house for the weekend. Sometimes it truly does take a village. I am so grateful for the village that I have.

I was shocked that I felt so dang good on day two. I still forced myself to stay in bed. Some of the things you forget: the sore nipples, the latching issues, and the not sleeping bit. The thing about doing the newborn baby thing multiple times was, my anxiety level went down. I knew all the struggles and challenges were going to be temporary. It made the postpartum period much more manageable. I'm so glad I chose to have a home birth. I truly believe that I would've delivered in the car on the way to the hospital if I had stuck with that choice. My pregnancy was rocky with all the prenatal bleeding, elevated test results, and anxiety, but my birth was the most uncomplicated delivery one could ask for. I'm so blessed. I'm also grateful that my home birth midwife welcomed me back and supported me through this journey. I thank her for seeing that three of my babies arrived earth-side safely.

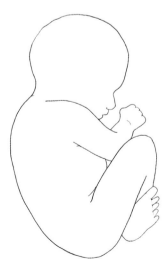

on Postpartum Depression

by Carrie Perry, *postpartum doula and mother*

Feeling overwhelmed is common. Skipping meals and lack of sleep can make things worse. Also know that postpartum mood disorders do not always manifest as "depression." Repetitive negative thoughts, obsessive-compulsive disorder, and anxiety are actually more common. If you are suffering, talk to somebody and get help sooner rather than later.

CALLING THE VILLAGE

Carriage House Birth's motto is "It takes a village." It is important to call upon your local village for support during your days newly postpartum. Don't be afraid to ask for what you need. Many people spend so much time planning for the birth that the postpartum period often gets neglected or not planned for at all. Communal living was the way of our ancestors, but it is not commonly practiced in our modern culture. We are often left alone feeling isolated and unsupported. Friends and family are often our first choice for support, but they are not always available or they may not live nearby. Reach out to your local community/village to inquire about postpartum doulas and/or lactation support. If your budget doesn't allow for these services, perhaps look into doulas-in-training or volunteer organizations that offer support postpartum. There are also local and online support groups for new parents. You don't have to walk this postpartum journey alone!

SLEEP

Oh sweet sleep, I miss you! The hardest part of becoming a new parent is the sleep deprivation. It's like going on a wild bender for days but without the drugs or the party. You never know beforehand what type of baby you will get, one who sleeps well or one who doesn't. I've had both types. I hate when people brag and say, "Well my little Johnny slept through the night since the day he was born . . . blah blah blah." They just happened to win the new parent lottery. You may win that lottery too. I hope you do. But if you don't, know that you are not alone. The good news is that newborns tend to sleep a lot. They may not sleep when you want them to, but they will be sleeping between fifteen and seventeen hours a day and waking every few hours.

Newborns don't seem to know the difference between night and day, which can result in super exhausted parents. I made a point to feed more frequently during the daylight hours, and it seemed to help them sleep in longer stretches at night. Now where is your baby going to sleep? A co-sleeper, your bed, a bassinet, or a nursery? In 2016, the American Academy of Pediatrics (AAP) recommended that infants share their parents' bedroom until at least six months of age to protect against sudden infant death syndrome (SIDS). I don't particularly like giving advice on where I think you should have your baby sleep. That's up to you. Just please do it safely.

I did something different with each of my children. After having two sets of twins, I had to do some form of gentle sleep training. Co-sleeping with four-month-old twins was becoming very dangerous and *not* very restful. I never was one for the cry-it-out approach. I couldn't do it. It went against my instincts. That said, I don't judge you for choosing whichever method helps you become a sane and well-rested parent. My last baby co-sleeps with me and probably will until she's thirty. No judgment.

Everyone will tell you what worked for them, and sleep experts make money on books that reveal the secret answer to getting your little ones to sleep. It is a hot topic among parents. Many suggest that letting your child cry it out is cruel and psychologically damaging. Others tend to every nighttime whimper and believe that parenting doesn't stop just because it's the middle of the night.

I am not an expert on infant sleep. I follow my instincts and my own need for sleep. Most of the sleep training techniques teach your newborn to fall asleep in their crib independently. If it feels wrong for your family, then it most likely is. Follow your instincts as a parent and don't be pushed into implementing a sleep training method because it worked for your neighbor, friend, or coworker. There is no one-size-fits-all trick to get babies to sleep peacefully. And they will eventually sleep. How many teenagers do you know who wake up at 5 a.m. and start bouncing off the walls? Not a single damn one, I bet.

SKIN-TO-SKIN CONTACT

I tell all my doula clients to plan on spending the first two weeks postpartum in bed skin to skin with their new babies. This is a great way to promote bonding with your newborn. That newborn baby smell is intoxicating, and you can feel the oxytocin flowing as you snuggle in bed. I swear this is why I'm addicted to having babies. It's these sweet moments that I spent postpartum skin to skin. This precious time spent bonding can reduce instances of postpartum depression. My babies slept better when they were laying skin to skin on my chest. Letting your baby sleep skin to skin on your chest can also allow you some time to rest and recover. It's survival in those first few weeks postpartum.

When you have a newborn, you will need a few safe places in your home to put your baby down. You may attempt to use the bathroom or take a shower without the baby in your arms. I can't tell you how many times I've gone to the bathroom with a baby on my lap or boob. It would be much nicer if you could put the baby down and know that the baby is safe. There are also times where you may need a few minutes to regroup and take a few deep breaths. Know that every single parent will at some point reach a state of complete frustration and despair when the baby becomes inconsolable.

NEWBORN FEEDING

Welcome to the world, little one! Now what do you do with this thing? Well, feed them. Newborns eat frequently and will hopefully regain their birth weight after around two weeks. All that eating may lead to spit-up and burping. Oh joy! It seems like some babies are just more prone to spitting up than others. There was a period of time with my first baby during which I couldn't leave the house without being spit up on. The nicer my outfit, the quicker she would spit up on me. Those burp cloths really came in handy.

CRYING

One of the most challenging things to a new parent is handling when your newborn baby cries. We are hardwired to our own baby's cry. The cry is going to affect you more than anyone who is supporting you postpartum. This is your little one's only form of communication. Some babies just cry more than others. Figuring out why your baby is crying can sometimes be confusing. Typically, it indicates hunger. Newborns have small stomachs and get hungry very frequently. If you are breast-feeding, this is called on-demand feeding. Even if you fed your baby fifteen minutes prior, there is a good chance that crying means they may be hungry again. Formula-fed babies are on a more consistent schedule and it's more like every two hours. It's okay if you want to offer the feeding a little bit earlier if your baby is fussing.

Your baby might also cry if they just want to be held, they're too cold or hot, they have a dirty diaper, or they're sleepy. If you check all these things and your baby is still fussy, there could be a chance that your baby is uncomfortable and perhaps has gas. You could try an infant massage with coconut oil every night after your baby's bath. I paid special attention to my babies' tummies and would bicycle their little legs and froggy them up toward their chest to help push out any gas. And remember that birth ball from labor? You can now bounce on your ball to help soothe a fussy baby postpartum. I loved bouncing and singing "You Are My Sunshine." It seems to do the trick.

COLIC

You may have heard the term *colic*. Colic is a blanket term for uncontrollable and often unexplained bouts of crying. Colic crying jags can last at least three hours, and the crying often turns to screaming. Causes have been linked to an immature digestive tract, infant acid reflux, food allergies, and overstimulation. Please reach out to your pediatrician if you suspect your little one has colic. I would also highly recommend seeking out emotional support. This can be especially hard on brand-new, sleep-deprived parents. Please go easy on yourself and know that colic is something that most babies grow out of as the weeks go by.

POOP

Those first few postpartum baby poops are called *meconium*. Meconium is a thick, greenish-black tar-like poo that can get stuck to your baby's bottom. After two to four days, your baby's poop starts to get lighter in color as it begins to mix with breastmilk or formula. An exclusively breastfed baby will start having yellow or greenish poop that looks like Dijon mustard and has an almost sweet smell. Formula-fed babies will have brownish poop with a toothpaste-like consistently and a pretty funky smell. I recommend rubbing coconut oil on your baby's bum after every poop so it's easier to clean the next diaper, and to prevent diaper rash. Always have a few extra outfits on hand, as accidents are frequent in those first few months.

BABY SKIN AND PIMPLES

Your sweet baby's skin is brand spanking new and sensitive. Her feet and hands may get super dry and peely, and newborn babies are prone to baby acne. Rash-like outbreaks are common on their cheeks and backs. These pesky pimples are caused by maternal hormones from when they were still tucked in your womb, and the pimples can last weeks to months. Time is really the only cure. I often would squirt the outbreaks with a little breastmilk. If you are breastfeeding, give it a try. Breastmilk cures everything, right?! As tempting as it may be, don't pick or squeeze their pimples. Avoid lotions and any scented soaps. Don't scrub, and pat dry after washing. Be patient. It just takes time for baby acne to clear.

UMBILICAL CORD

The umbilical cord stump is a powerful reminder of the physical connection you once had to your baby. Your baby's stump needs to be kept dry in those first few days postpartum until it falls off. This can take anywhere from one to two weeks. Please don't pick at it like a scab. There can be a little blood when it falls off. Check in with your pediatrician if there is any pus and/or if the surrounding area becomes swollen and red.

Recommended umbilical cord care always seems to be changing. In the past, you were supposed to use rubbing alcohol to clean the umbilical cord site. Now pediatricians recommend leaving it completely alone to heal. A few natural remedies to help aid healing are breastmilk and/or goldenseal powder. Breastmilk has antibodies and antibacterial properties that can prevent infection. I love this magical elixir! Goldenseal powder has been recommended by midwives for many years to aid in healing the umbilical stump. This herb is said to speed the healing process considerably. You should check in to see what your care provider suggests.

SWADDLING

The swaddle can either be an absolute lifesaver or a torture device, depending on your baby. Most babies tend to like being snuggled up tight just like they were back in the womb. I like to call it *the baby burrito* or *the glowworm*. If your baby is born in the hospital, the nurses love to swaddle because it makes their job a bit easier. It makes for fewer crying babies for them to juggle. When supporting my doula clients in the hospital, I tend to unwrap the baby and make sure baby is skin to skin on the parents as much as possible, at least during the first few days outside of the womb. Not many people sleep well during their hospital stay. They wake you up every hour or so to check on your vitals and the baby. You typically arrive home utterly exhausted and desperate for sleep. The swaddle keeps your baby asleep for longer stretches because they don't wake themself up with their own startle reflex. The AAP states that swaddling, if used correctly, can be an effective method to calm your baby and promote sleep.

Babies can be swaddled up to around five to six months old. Once your babe starts to bust out of the swaddle, it may become a hazard. I don't think I would have survived twins twice if it weren't for swaddling, while my singletons hated the swaddle with a passion and preferred being skin to skin on my warm chest or in a baby carrier. This is another parenting tool that you may or may not use for your baby. It's nice to know you have some options that may assist you on your parenting journey.

HOW TO SWADDLE

First you need to select something to swaddle with. My favorites are muslin swaddle blankets. They are multipurpose and can be used as blankets, spit rags, and coverage from the sun. They are great for every season because they are breathable. Babies can overheat in an extremely thick blanket.

- Start by laying your blanket down in a diamond shape on a flat surface.
- Fold the top corner down. Place your baby on the blanket, lining up the baby's neck on the fold.
- Next hold your babe's right arm down by his side and pull the left corner of the swaddle over his right arm and across his body. Securely tuck the corner under his left arm and back.
- Hold down your babe's left arm and pull up the bottom of the diamond over his left shoulder. To finish up and enter glow-worm status, bring the right corner across the front of your baby and wrap the corner around to the back.

BABYWEARING

Babywearing is a huge lifesaver for a new parent. It is the practice of wearing your baby in a carrier or a sling, and it is by no means a new innovation. Parents have been wearing babies for many centuries all around the world. When none of your tricks works to soothe your fussy baby, put them in a carrier. Within minutes, the movement and the closeness to your heartbeat will lull them to sleep. It's the only way many parents are able to do anything for the first three months. My first baby hated being out of my arms, so the carrier was a game-changing solution.

BATHING

When should you give your newborn her first bath? The World Health Organization strongly recommends delaying a bath for at least twenty-four hours post-delivery. Many hospitals have a different policy, though, so be sure to ask. Delaying the bath and keeping your baby in skin-to-skin contact with you for the first twenty-four hours will help keep her warm. Another plus for delaying the first bath is that babies are born covered in vernix. Vernix is a frosting-like coating on your baby's skin that protects her from bacterial infections. Vernix is also a natural moisturizer and insulator for your baby's newly exposed skin. As the birth doula, I am often tempted to use baby vernix for undereye cream. Don't worry, I'll never do it, but I'd be lying if I said that I've never thought about it. Instead of wiping the vernix off your baby, rub it in.

Believe it or not, your newborn really doesn't need frequent baths. Just be mindful of keeping the diaper area clean. Until they're crawling around on the floor, a few baths a week should be sufficient. Too many baths can dry out sensitive newborn skin.

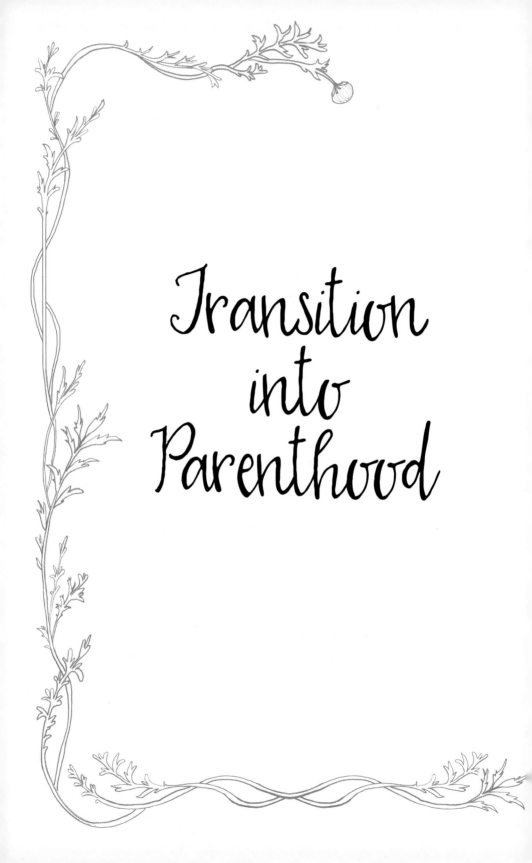

Transition into Parenthood

THE JOURNEY TO PARENTHOOD IS A WILDLY TRANSFOR-
mative experience. Nothing else in life pushes the bounds of love and
struggle in quite the same ways. As new parents, you are going to screw
up constantly. Be easy on yourself and remember that you get to try again
every day.

EMBRACING CHAOS

The words *embracing chaos* have become a bit of a motto for me. I am a
very steady Taurus through and through. I like my feet grounded firmly
in the earth. Having all these kids has definitely taught me to surrender
and embrace chaos. That doesn't mean there can't be an outline drawn
around the chaos to help it feel contained and much more manageable.
The one thing that you can control is how you feel about any given
situation. If you decide no matter what the outcome is that you are going
to remain positive, you will have a positive experience. If you give in to
fear and despair, your experience is going to be negative and filled with
fear. The older I get and the more babies I have, the more I trust the flow
of things. I am a very active participant in life, but I will often choose to
sit back and go along for the ride when I can't "control" a situation. All of
this relates to pregnancy, childbirth, and parenting.

I have a vivid memory of going to the grocery store with my newborn twins, my two-year-old twins, and my five-year-old. I had to pull the
double stroller behind me as I pushed the shopping cart in front of me
while I made sure the two-year-olds were not running through the aisles.
Before I went inside, I gave myself a pep talk. I tried to make it feel like a
game or a challenge. I decided to laugh that day instead of cry because it
was starting to feel crushingly overwhelming. Let me tell you, it worked.
I tried to let things roll off me instead of feeling held back. How I must
have looked in the parking lot patting myself on the back and cracking
jokes with my kids!

on Parenting

by Elizabeth Bachner, *midwife and owner of GraceFull Birth*

There is no formula or technique that can guarantee a specific experience or outcome, for we are not in control, which is the first lesson in parenting. The second lesson is in the trusting of the process. Each birth is a journey of our own creation in which spirit offers up life lessons to be learned on the wings of god's angels, our master teachers, the children we are birthing. No matter what your birth looks like, it is always guided by Grace, which can be seen with a shift in perspective, from the limited view of victim and victor into one of embodied compassion and love, for ourselves and others, which is the soul's purpose as to why we are here.

Embracing chaos also reminds me of a doula client of mine who had a birth outcome that was very far from what she was hoping for. She beautifully embraced chaos and went along for the ride. She taught me that you can have a "traumatic" birth but still have it be beautiful and ceremonious. I'll never forget the look in her eyes as she beamed at her baby. She chose love, and so love won that day.

SIBLINGS

Introducing your new baby to your other children may be challenging, depending on the child. But with good reason! Imagine this: Your partner (if you have one) comes home and tells you that he or she found another wife or husband that you're going to love. He or she will be moving in with you in nine months, and you have absolutely no say in the matter.

Go easy with them. Let them know that it's okay to have all different types of feelings surrounding the arrival of a new baby. Hold space for them to process their feelings. Talk about the baby coming and help them form a relationship early on. Retelling their own baby stories may help them become more familiar with a new baby. When the baby arrives, you can make them feel important by including them in the newborn care. Have them fetch diapers or pick out outfits. During breastfeeding or bottle feeding, the older sibling may start to feel excluded. A great option is to include them by inviting them to sit beside you.

As a parent, you need to know that it is completely possible to love multiple children. Your heart just keeps getting bigger.

INTRODUCING PETS

I am an animal lover. My dogs were my first babies. They taught me about being responsible for another living thing. Many clients I work with fear the reaction their pets may have to the introduction of a new baby. My dog was aware something was about to change during my pregnancy. She followed me everywhere and didn't allow anyone in the house unannounced. She nearly attacked the mailman for getting too close to me.

Animals tend to mirror our behavior. Make an effort to be extra calm and firm around your dog. Let her know that you are the leader of the pack. Once the baby is born, you can bring a receiving blanket with the baby's scent home to the dog. Allow the dog to become familiar with the baby's scent before being introduced. A client of mine was so concerned about her beloved pet's potential negative reaction to the new baby that she hired an animal trainer/behaviorist. They helped this family reduce anxiety and develop a game plan for the transition. Luckily their pooch got used to the new addition without any major hiccups. My biggest piece of advice is to never leave your dog around your baby unsupervised. Once babies start crawling, they can poke eyes and yank tails.

Even the nicest of pups can turn if provoked. Teach your baby to handle animals gently.

Cats, unfortunately, are a little bit more of a wild card. You can use the receiving blanket to get your cat familiar with your newborn baby's smell. I've had numerous cats through the years, and all of them were fine, except one. This cat seemed to snap and turned aggressive toward my babies. I was fortunate enough to be able to re-home him to a child-free home. Another thing to watch out for is the cat trying to jump into the crib and sleep with the baby. A cat using the litter box and then trying to sleep next to your baby is not a good idea. They make crib tents to keep curious cats out.

Good luck introducing your pets to your new baby. Hopefully you will all find your groove and become one big happy family.

SOCIAL LIFE

Pre-babies, I had a very active social life. I was not prepared for the huge lifestyle shift of becoming a parent. During pregnancy, a few of my friends slipped away. After I gave birth to my first daughter, a bunch more disappeared. The socializing that I found to be so important pre-baby was not very significant compared to my new role as a mother. Everything in my life paled in comparison to my daughter. My life had a meaning that I never knew was missing. Many first-time parents are under the illusion that things are not going to change as drastically as they do. Many believe that the baby is going to adapt to their lifestyle. It's the opposite. You completely change everything to adapt to your new baby.

SEX

The rule is to wait six weeks (or less if your bleeding stops sooner) to resume sex so that your body can heal completely. The problem that remains is that you may be completely touched out from caring for a newborn 24/7. Breastfeeding hormones can also greatly reduce your sex drive. Sleep and food become the new sex. Your partner may be ready and feel hurt by this shift in priorities. Be sure to find other ways to show your love and appreciation. Cuddling, napping together, and spending time together as a family can help keep that intimate connection with your partner. Having a baby with someone may also make you fall deeper in love with them (or want to leave them). On the opposite end of the spectrum, you may be one of those people who can't wait for that six-week mark to arrive. Props to you!

GRATITUDE

Thank you, universe, for the gift of being a mother to healthy children. Thank you for my amazing and supportive partner. Thank you for allowing me to support, inform, and hold space for expecting families during their childbearing journey. It's an honor beyond my wildest dreams.

What are you grateful for? How often do you stop to appreciate what you have in life instead of what you don't have? Being a new parent is hard. Remembering to be grateful will make your hardest parenting struggles seem manageable. It's so easy to get caught up in the everyday stresses of being a parent that you don't stop and smell the roses. You may find yourself complaining way too often about that never-ending pile of laundry, your messy house, lack of money, lack of time, lack of sleep . . . and the list drags on. The glass feels half empty sometimes. But gratitude is what gets poured into that glass to make it half full.

I want my children to be grateful and empathetic souls. To teach them this, we must model that behavior. We are their role models and guides on this journey.

Here are some ways to incorporate gratitude into your daily life:

○ Work on relaxing and living in the moment. When we are stressed out and anxious, it's almost impossible to express gratitude.

○ Choose to be grateful.

○ Stop complaining. Treat yourself to a one-day, one-week, or two-week No Complaining Challenge. It's easier said than done. It's a great exercise to be mindful of your negative thoughts.

○ At dinner or bedtime, have everyone list one or two good things that happened during the day. Get in the habit of doing this every day. Eventually you will be looking for the good in every situation.

○ Give back. Volunteer at a local charity. Sweep or rake leaves for your elderly neighbor or bring flowers to a friend. Do something nice for someone else.

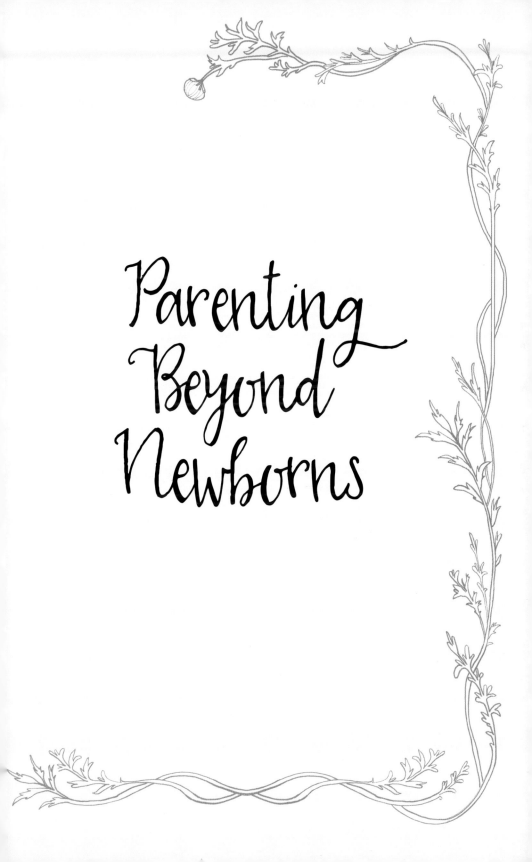

Parenting Beyond Newborns

BECOMING A PARENT WAS THE HARDEST THING THAT I
have ever done in my life. The crushing responsibility of keeping my
child alive and safe from harm was no joke. The beauty of this whole
parenting gig is that there are also many rewards. Here are a few parenting tips that can help you navigate your early days and years in
new parenthood.

- Babies will eventually sleep. Really, they will. Everyone is quick to
  give you advice and/or tips on getting your baby to sleep. Trust your
  gut and know that sleep deprivation is just a phase of this new parenting journey.

- Random playground parents can be extremely judgmental. It can
  sometimes be a drama-filled high school flashback on the playground.
  I enjoy making new friends and will often strike up a casual conversation. I typically get the once-over twice. Really? I just wanted to
  talk to another adult. I thought that by becoming a mommy I joined a
  sorority of sisterhood created by the bonds of motherhood!

- No one will ever understand your situation completely. Friends and
  family members may get a glimpse of your beautiful madhouse, but
  you're left alone (maybe with a partner) to really understand the mag-
  nitude of this childbearing journey. Having seven children, this really
  resonates with me.

- You will never *need* to buy a new pair of high heels again. Unless, of
  course, you want to. I wear heels once a year, maybe. Wearing pumps
  and pushing a double stroller looks uncomfortable.

- You may really love being a parent. I was worried that I got myself into
  a real mess of butt-wiping and wrangling screaming, snot-nosed kids.
  I did, and I'm so lucky and grateful for it. My life is full. Your baby can
  bring you a sense of joy that is beyond comprehension.

SURVIVING TODDLERS

In my house, we often have what I call *the twin tantrum*. It's two scream-ing and crying little monsters. Sometimes I get really lucky and all of my children will join in on the fun. Energy is infectious! I have learned a few things to help make these episodes less frequent and much more man-ageable. I will try to share with you some of the things that have worked for us. Each child is different, so these tips may not apply to everyone. I don't have a specific style of parenting; I really don't believe that one style/approach to parenting can apply to every child. They are all unique.

Breathe. Pause. Take really deep breaths to help remain calm. Toddlers can sense when you are getting aggravated and will use it against you. The more worked up you get, the more they work you. As silly as it sounds, counting to ten in your head works wonders.

Don't yell. I know this one can be hard, because I occasionally snap and yell. No one is perfect, and I understand what it's like to reach your boil-ing point. Yelling will often extend the duration of the tantrum and just scare the crap out of your toddler.

Don't hit your kids. Really, what good comes out of spanking your kid? I'm not trying to be judgmental, but learning a nonviolent approach to parenting will benefit you and your child immensely. Getting the urge to smack them is normal. Trust me, I would often like to. But I don't, and I never will. There are other effective ways to guide your children.

Don't pacify the situation. I know sometimes it would be easier to give them what they want so they stop shrieking, but it only makes them think that these tantrums will work to get them what they want. My friend once said, "I don't negotiate with terrorists." Love this. Be strong.

Don't be afraid to parent your kids. Your kids may not like you sometimes, but so what? You will do them a huge disservice by just being their friend. Set boundaries and teach them to respect you and other global citizens. Would you let another grown-up talk to you the way your toddler does? I personally have a hard time being friends with adults who are spoiled brats with no boundaries. I'm trying hard to ensure that my kids won't be narcissists when they grow up.

Time-outs work for most kids. If time-outs don't work, try putting their favorite toy or game in time out. I know there are some heated debates on whether this is a good technique or not, but it works in my house, so I do it.

Redirect the tantrum. Sometimes I will start dancing or laughing wildly during one of their tantrums, and they will often stop, a bit confused. Either way, the bad behavior or fit stops. Well, not always, but it makes me laugh to act the fool and I'm less angry while dealing with their multiple meltdowns.

Lastly, make sure you give your kids lots of positive reinforcement. On days that we play together tons and I have fewer chores around the house, they seem a lot happier. With a large family, my kids are always competing for my attention. I really work hard to reward good behavior in our house.

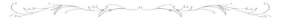

Don't be afraid to parent your kids.
Your kids may not like you sometimes,
but so what? You will do them a huge
disservice by just being their friend.
Set boundaries.

REFERENCES

The Cochrane Database of Systematic Reviews

The World Health Organization (WHO)

American Congress of Obstetrics and Gynecologists (ACOG)

The Journal of Obstetrics and Gynecology

U.S. Department of Health and Human Services

Environmental Working Group (EWG)

Cambridge Dictionary

Centers for Disease Control and Prevention (CDC)

American Academy of Anesthesiologists

The Lamaze Method

HypnoBirthing

Doula Organization of North America (DONA)

The Bradley Method of Natural Childbirth

The American Academy of Pediatrics

Carriage House Birth

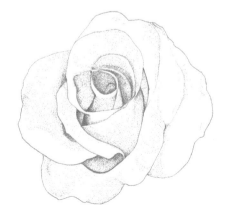

EXPERT BIOS

Elizabeth Bachner, LM, CPM, and L.Ac is the creator of the Los Angeles–based environmentally respectful birthing center *GraceFull Birthing,* where she is the clinic director and a practicing midwife. Elizabeth co-facilitates childbirth education classes and various workshops.
Website: www.gracefull.com
Instagram: gracefullbirth

Robin Rose Bennett is an herbalist, wisewoman, teacher, and green witch. She is the author of *Ocean and Moon* meditation CDs and two books, *Healing Magic: A Green Witch Guidebook to Conscious Living* and *The Gift of Healing Herbs.*
Website: www.robinrosebennett.com

Carriage House Birth strives to provide pregnant people with a family system. The success of their model is grounded in the cultivation of relationships among the members of their doula collective. They believe that it is imperative for birth doulas, postpartum doulas, and body workers to all interact with each other so that they feel comfortable with calling on one another for support. Domino Kirke, Samantha Huggins, and Lindsey Bliss are the triad of mothers and birth doulas who own and run Carriage House Birth. Their village of support is currently in New York City and Los Angeles and is growing by the day.

Carriage House Birth has served over 1,500 families in New York and Los Angeles since 2011 with birth and postpartum support, breastfeeding/infant feeding support, childbirth education, and more.
Website: www.carriagehousebirth.com
Instagram: carriagehousebirth
Email: info@carriagehousebirth.com

LaShanda Dandrich is an International Board Certified Lactation Consultant (IBCLC), a postpartum doula, and a mother. She is the founder of the Uptown Village Co-op located in Harlem, New York City, and is available for lactation consultant home visits.
Website: www.UptownVillage.coop
Email: UptownVillageLC@gmail.com

Deborah Hanekamp (aka Mama Medicine) is a seeress carrying over seventeen years in the healing arts. She is an initiated Amazonian shaman, reiki master, and yogini. Guided by the present moment, Deborah has facilitated medicine readings and medicine reading ceremonies all over the world. Her work has been featured in *Vogue*, the *New York Times*, and *Marie Claire* magazine. To book a session, email appointments@mama-medicine.nyc or call 212-226-1714.
Website: www.mamamedicine.nyc
Instagram: mamamedicine

Samantha Huggins is a founder and co-director of Carriage House Birth, a CHB-certified intuitive birth doula, a mother of two kids, a lactation counselor, a childbirth educator, and co-founder of The Code, a radical sex education program for tweens.
Website: www.carriagehousebirth.com and www.thekidcode.org
Instagram: the_kidcode

Miracle Mattie was a massage therapist, an herbalist, a mother, a grandmother, and a great-grandmother. She has left us earth-side but her wisdom and love still remain.

Shafia M. Monroe, DEM, CDT, and MPH, is the founder of the International Center for Traditional Childbearing (ICTC) and community activist devoted to infant mortality prevention, breastfeeding promotion, and increasing the number of midwives of color. In addition to being a certified midwife by the Massachusetts Midwives Alliance, she is also a childbirth educator, a doula trainer, and the mother of seven children.

Website: www.shafiamonroe.com
Email: shafia@shafiamonroe.com

Carrie Perry is a mother of two, a lactation counselor, and a postpartum doula in Brooklyn, New York.
Website: www.carriagehousebirth.com

Jessica Prescott is a mama, writer, and photographer of the vegan blog *Wholy Goodness*. She is also the author of the book *Vegan Goodness: Delicious Plant-Based Recipes That Can Be Enjoyed by Anyone.*
Website: www.wholygoodness.com
Instagram: wholygoodness

Tara Stiles is a mother, a yoga instructor, an author, and the founder of Strala Yoga. Tara created Strala by drawing on her background in classical ballet and choreography, as well as her longtime personal practice in yoga. She collaborated with Reebok to create the Reebok Yoga lifestyle line, and she has authored several best-selling books, including *Yoga Cures, Make Your Own Rules Cookbook*, and *Strala Yoga*, all translated and published in many languages.
Website: www.stralayoga.com and www.tarastiles.com
Instagram: tarastiles

Loveday Why is a writer, healer, coach, and founder of the healthy eating and lifestyle blog *Wild & Good*.
Website: www.wild-and-good.com
Instagram: wild_and_good

Dr. Jessica Zucker is a Los Angeles–based psychologist and writer specializing in women's reproductive and maternal mental health. She is also the creator of the #IHadAMiscarriage campaign.
Website: www.drjessicazucker.com
Instagram: ihadamiscarriage

FINDING A CARE PROVIDER

It's important to interview potential care providers to make sure they practice evidence-based care and that they're an appropriate fit for you. Use the following list as a guide, or photocopy it and fill in the answers. See "Choosing Your Care Provider," beginning on page 72, for more information.

Do you practice evidence-based care?

_____

_____

What are your philosophies surrounding pregnancy, labor, and childbirth?

_____

_____

What is your cesarean rate? (A lower rate is typically better, as most people are hoping to avoid a surgical delivery. If you are planning a cesarean, there's no need to be concerned; the cesarean rate is at an all-time high, so most practices are very experienced.)

_____

_____

Do you routinely induce clients at a certain number of weeks pregnant?

_____

_____

Do you routinely cut episiotomies? (An episiotomy is a surgical cut in the perineum, the area between the vagina and the anus, made to enlarge the vaginal opening for delivery. This used to be a routine procedure many years ago and is now only used in certain cases.)

_____

_____

Do you routinely rupture the bag of waters?

_____

_____

What other standard routine practices should I expect?

_____

_____

Who will be my care provider if you are not on call for my delivery?

_____

_____

How do you feel about doulas?

_____

_____

Do you have a time limit on the length of labor?

_____

_____

Can I room in with my baby (meaning have your baby stay in your room as opposed to the nursery)?

_____

_____

Is the hospital baby/family friendly?

_____

_____

ACKNOWLEDGMENTS

I would like to thank Samantha Huggins, Domino Kirke, The Carriage House Birth Community, Deborah Hanekamp, Tara Stiles, LaShanda Dandrich, Elizabeth Bachner, Robin Rose Bennet, Shafia Monroe, Jessica Prescott, Jessica Zucker, Carrie Perry, and my midwife, Cara Muhlhan.

ABOUT THE ILLUSTRATOR

Stepha is a doula, artist, counselor, mom, and owner of The Language of Birth, a platform dedicated to exploring how we talk about birth today and how birth talks to us. The all-encompassing lens in which she approaches this field is reflected in her illustrations: that spirited intersection of the plant and human world, holding timeless the cycles which seek to seed, to be born, to sprout, to grow, to wither and then die away. Stepha knows birth speaks in a similar power of survival and of magic.

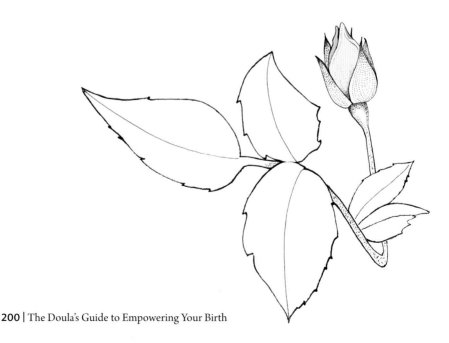

ABOUT THE AUTHOR

Lindsey Bliss is the co-director of Brooklyn's Carriage House Birth, a collective of birth workers that provide doula support and education for families pre-conception though their childbearing journeys. She is a birth doula, and mother of seven. Trained by DONA (Doulas of North America) and Carriage House Birth certified, Lindsey is greatly sought after and considered to be a multiples expert after giving birth and breast-feeding two consecutive sets of twins.

Her interest in childbirth began at an early age. Present while her mother taught childbirth education classes at their home, Lindsey was able to state, identify, and point out a uterus on a natal chart at the age of two and a half. Fast-forward to the present, Lindsey takes her role as a birth doula and childbirth educator with serious passion and commitment. Her mission is to hold space or offer gentle, nonjudgmental guidance and support for expectant families through education and informed decision making. Being prepared and knowing what options are available increase the likelihood of an amazing birth. Lindsey facilitates that process, giving people the tools and inspiration to empower themselves. Her unwavering support and gentle guidance have benefited more than two hundred families. Lindsey supports first-time parents, multiparas, single parents, LGBTQ families, twin births, medicated and nonmedicated vaginal births, cesarean births, and VBACs.

INDEX

Also available from
The Harvard Common Press

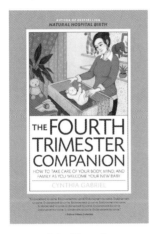

The Fourth
Trimester Companion
978-1-55832-887-7

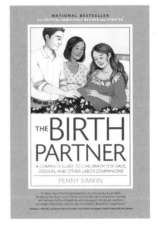

The Birth Partner, 4th Edition
978-1-55832-880-8

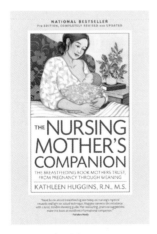

The Nursing
Mother's Companion
978-1-55832-882-2

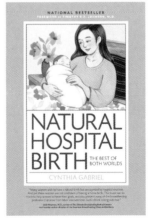

Natural Hospital Birth
978-1-55832-881-5